General and Systematic Veterinary Virology

General and Systematic Veterinary Virology

Dr. (Mrs.) Varsha Sharma, Ph.D.
Professor and Head
Veterinary Microbiology, College of Veterinary
Science and Animal Husbandry, Jabalpur (M.P.)

Dr. (Mrs.) Anju Nayak
Associate Professor
Veterinary Microbiology, College of Veterinary
Science and Animal Husbandry, Jabalpur (M.P.)

Dr. Vandana Gupta
Assistant Professor in the Department of Veterinary
Microbiology, Veterinary College, Rewa

Dr. Sanjay Kumar Shukla
Assistant Professor in the Department of Veterinary
College of Veterinary Science & A.H., J.N.K.V.V., Jabalpur

Dr. Poonam Shakya
Assistant Professor
Department of Veterinary Microbiology
Veterinary College, Jabalpur

Dr. Ajay Rai
Assistant Professor
Department of Veterinary Microbiology, College of Veterinary
Science and Animal Husbandry, Jabalpur (M.P.)

SSPH

SATISH SERIAL PUBLISHING HOUSE
403, Express Tower, Commercial Complex
Azadpur, Delhi-110033 (India)
Phone : 011-27672852, Fax : 91-11-27672046
e-mail : info@satishserial.com, hkjain1975@yahoo.com
Website : www.satishserial.com

Published by :

SATISH SERIAL PUBLISHING HOUSE
403, Express Tower, Commercial Complex, Azadpur, Delhi-110033 (INDIA)
Phone : 011-27672852 Fax : 91-11-27672046
E-mail : info@satishserial.com, hkjain1975@yahoo.com

ISBN 978-93-88020-36-7

Composed, Designed & Printed in India

About the Authors

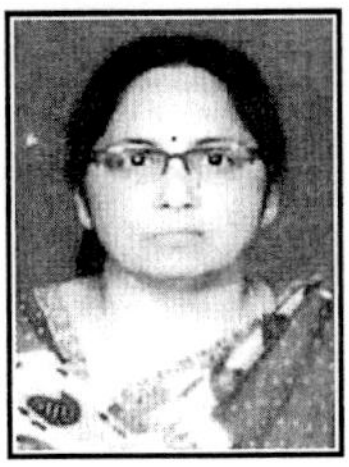

Dr. (Mrs.) Varsha Sharma Ph.D., is at presently working as Professor and Head Veterinary Microbiology, College of Veterinary Science and Animal Husbandry, Jabalpur (M.P.) She has also served as Veterinary Assistant Surgeon in M.P. State Services for 4 years and 23 years experience in teaching, research and extension. Dr. Sharma has pursued her B.V.Sc. & A.H. and M.V.Sc. & A.H. in Veterinary Microbiology from College of Veterinary Science and A.H., JNKVV, Jabalpur. She has guided several students in Microbiology from Veterinary and general stream of various universities. She has published about 01 Technical Bulletin, 03 practical Manuals, 03 Review articles, 75 Research articles, about 115 Abstracts and 25 Popular articles and leaflets.

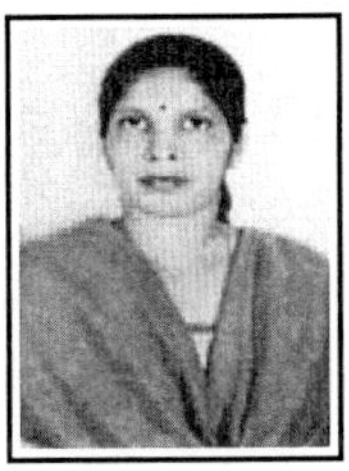

Dr. (Mrs.) Anju Nayak, is at present working as Associate Professor, Veterinary Microbiology, College of Veterinary Science and Animal Husbandry, Jabalpur (M.P.) She has a vast experience of veterinary extension, research and teaching. She is the recipient of University Gold Medal for undergraduate programme from I.G.K.V.V., Raipur (C.G.). She did her post graduation with specialization in Veterinary Immunology from Indian Veterinary Research Institute. She has pursued her Ph.D. from College of Veterinary Science and A.H., JNKVV, Jabalpur. She has a number of research and popular articles to her credit.

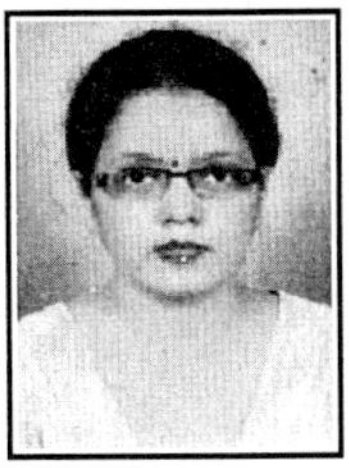

Dr. Vandana Gupta is working in the capacity of Assistant Professor in the Department of Veterinary Microbiology, Veterinary College, Rewa. She has done her Masters in Veterinary Microbiology from Anand Agricultural University, Anand. At present, pursuing her Ph.D. in Veterinary Virology, from Department of Veterinary Microbiology, Veterinary College, Jabalpur. She holds 11 years experience in teaching and research. She has bagged National awards and fellowships and has a number of research and popular articles to her credit.

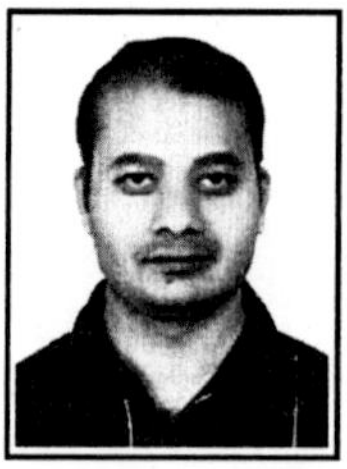

Dr. Sanjay Kumar Shukla is graduated from College of Veterinary Science & A.H., J.N.K.V.V., Jabalpur in 2007 and post graduate in Veterinary Microbiology, 2009 with same university. He is presently working as Assistant Professor/Scientist in the Department of Veterinary Microbiology, C.V.Sc. & A.H., N.D.V.S.U. Jabalpur (M.P.), India. He is having 8 years teaching/ research/extension experience. He has published total 25 Research, Review and Popular Articles. He has got "Fellowship for Training of Young Scientist "by M.P. Council of Science & Technology (M.P.C.S.T.), Bhopal (M.P.).

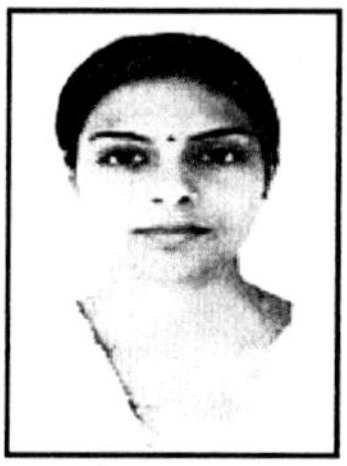

Dr. Poonam Shakya is working in the capacity of Assistant Professor in the Department of Veterinary Microbiology, Veterinary College, Jabalpur. She completed her Bachelor's and Master's degree from Veterinary College Mhow and grabbed the University Gold Medal. At present, she is pursuing her Ph.D. in Veterinary Microbiology, from Department of Veterinary Microbiology, Jabalpur. She has worked as Veterinary Assistant Surgeon for 4 years and holds 6 years of experience in teaching and research. She has published a number of research articles in various national and international journals as well as popular and extension articles in magazines and newspapers.

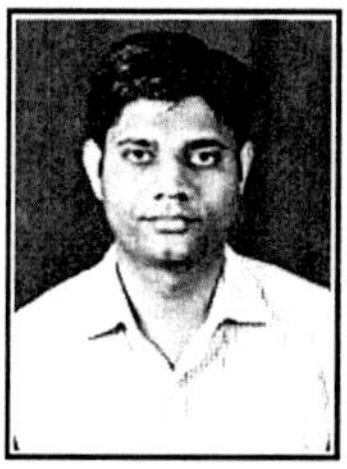

Dr. Ajay Rai has been working as Assistant Professor in the Department of Veterinary Microbiology, College of Veterinary Science and Animal Husbandry, Jabalpur (M.P.) since 2015. He has graduated from College of Veterinary Science and Animal Husbandry, Mhow (M.P.) in 2010. He has completed his Master's in Veterinary Bacteriology from Indian Veterinary Research Institute, Izatnagar, Bareilly (U.P.) in 2012. He holds 6 years experience in Research and Teaching. He has fellowships and number of research, review and popular articles to his credit.

नानाजी देशमुख पशुचिकित्सा विज्ञान विश्वविद्यालय, जबलपुर
आई/4–आई 4 के, लाला लाजपत राय वार्ड (वार्ड 45), साउथ सिविल लाईन्स
जबलपुर 482001 (म.प्र.) भारत
Nanaji Deshmukh Veterinary Science University, Jabalpur
I/4 -I/4K, Lala Lajpat Rai Ward (Ward 45), South Civil Lines,
Jabalpur 482001, (M.P.) India
(Established by MP Act No. 16 of 2009)

प्रो. (डॉ.) प्रयाग दत्त जुयाल
कुलपति
Prof. (Dr.) Prayag Dutt Juyal
Vice Chanellor

Phone cum Fax : 0761-2678007 (O)
Mobile No.: 9522581917
Email: vcnduvs@gmail.com
website:www.ndvsu.org

FOREWORD

This is a matter of immense pleasure that Professor(s) of Department of Veterinary Microbiology, College of Veterinary Science and Animal Husbandry, Nanaji Deshmukh Veterinary Science University Jabalpur, Dr. Varsha Sharma, Dr. Anju Nayak, Dr Vandana Gupta, Dr. Sanjay Kumar Shukla, Dr. Poonam Shakya and Dr. Ajay Rai have published the scientific Manual on "General and Systematic Veterinary Virology". This manual is based on new curriculum of VCI for student's benefits.

I hope that this manual would be very beneficial for undergraduate students.

(P.D. Juyal)
Vice Chancellor
NDVSU, Jabalpur (MP)

Contents

About the Authors .... *v*
Foreword .... *vii*
Preface .... *ix*

Laboratory Rules 1

1. Orientation to a Virology Laboratory 5
2. Collection, Preservation, Transport of Samples and their Processing in Virology Laboratory 15
3. Isolation of Viruses 25
4. Preparation of Media and Reagents for Cell Culture 45
5. Subculture and Maintenance of Continuous Cell Lines 55
6. Quantitation of Cells by Viable Cell Counts in a Haemocytometer 59
7. Cryopreservation and Recovery of Cell Cultures 63
8. Preparation of Primary Cell Culture 65
9. Demonstration of Cytopathic Effect by Viruses in Cell Culture 69
10. Demonstration of Titration of Virus by $TCID_{50}$ and Plaque Assay in Cell Cultures 71
11. Demonstration of Neutralizing Antibodies by Serum Neutralization Test in Cell Culture 83
12. Agar Gel Precipitation Test for Detection of Virus Infection 87
13. Titration of New Castle Disease Virus by Haemagglutination Test 89
14. Haemagglutination Inhibition Test for Detection of Antibodies to New Castle Disease Virus 91
15. ELISA for Detection of Viral Antigen and Antibodies 93
16. Molecular Techniques for Viral Disease Diagnosis 99

Laboratory Rules

1. Attendance in laboratory is mandatory. Please be on time.
2. Wear a lab coat or apron-they are easier to sterilize than your clothing, if you spill a culture or staining reagents.
3. No eating or drinking in lab.
4. Only mechanical pipetting no mouth pipetting. Never lick your fingers, or put your fingers in your mouth.
5. Treat every organism as a potential pathogen.
6. Consider all chemicals hazardous. Never taste any chemical or inhale any vapour.
7. Treat spilled cultures with disinfectant before cleaning them up.
8. No Gadgets are allowed in the lab.
9. All cultures, whether in test tubes or petri plates, should be labelled with your name or initials, the date, and the name of the organism. Plates can be written on directly-always on the bottom of the plate. Permanent markers designated only for laboratory use must be used to label cultures.
10. Most microbial cultures will be inoculated using a sterile loop or needle; once the transfer is complete the loop or needle should be sterilized again. Liquid cultures should be transferred using a sterile pipette and mechanical pipetting apparatus.
11. All test tubes should be placed in a rack before transporting them from one area of the lab to another. All lids on all test tubes must be secure.
12. All disposable microbiological waste should be discarded in the BIOHAZARD bag. Used test tubes should be placed in the designated pan to be autoclaved and cleaned. Used pipettes should be placed immediately into the provided waste container.

Do not place any hazardous or infectious materials in the regular trash. Do not place any hazardous or infectious materials in the sink.

13. Practice good aseptic technique by performing the following at the end of each lab exercise:
    a) Remove gloves inside out and place them in the biohazard bag.
    b) Remove lab coats or aprons, fold them inside out, and place them in the assigned drawer.
    c) Decontaminate your work bench by applying an antiseptic wash.
    d) Wash your hands thoroughly.
    e) Do not write in your lab manual or notebook until after you have removed your gloves and apron and washed your hands.
14. All reagents, stains and other equipments should be returned to their original place at the end of the laboratory period.

Biosafety Guidelines & Biosafety Levels

The four basic routes of exposure to micro-organisms are:

1. **Contact** with skin and mucous membranes-It can be minimized by wearing aprons, gloves, etc.
2. **Ingestion**-It can be minimized by prohibiting eating and drinking.
3. **Inhalation**-It can be minimized by adopting measures which decrease the likelihood of generating aerosols (infected airborne droplets).
4. **Inoculation**-It can be minimized by initiating rigid protocols for the use and disposal of sharp needles, slides, glass, etc.

Biosafety Levels (BSL)

Micro-organisms are divided into 4 Biosafety Levels (BSL) by the Centers for Disease Control and prevention.

BSL 1 organisms are well–characterized strains of micro-organisms not known to cause disease in healthy human adults.

Precautions in BSL-1 labs include general lab safety rules. Some examples of BSL-1 organisms–non-pathogenic strains of *Bacillus stearothermophilus, Bacillus subtilis, Enterobacter aerogenes, Enterobacter cloacae, Escherichia coli, Staphylococcus epidermidis, Streptococcus bovis, Streptococcus mutans,* etc.

BSL-2 organisms are moderate–risk micro-organisms that are associated with less serious human diseases whose potential for transmission is limited and a proven treatment for the disease exists. Many BSL-2 pathogens are opportunistic, meaning they don't ordinarily cause disease in healthy human adults, but may cause disease in children and immuno-compromised adults. Additional precautions in BSL-2 labs include using personal protective equipment (PPE), such as disposable gloves and lab coats and limiting lab access to trained individuals. Some examples of BSL-2 organisms include *Bacillus cereus,Edwardsiella tarda, Enterococcus faecalis, Klebsiella pneumoniae, Proteus mirabilis, Proteus vulgaris, Pseudomonas aeruginosa, Salmonella* Typhimurium, *Salmonella choleraesuis, Staphylococcus aureus, Streptococcus agalactiae, Streptococcus pyogenes, Streptococcus equi, Streptococcus equi subspecies zooepidemicus,* Adenoviruses, Poliovirus, Coxsackievirus, Hepatitis viruses, Toxoplasma and Leishmania, etc.

BSL-3 organisms are high risk micro organisms with true potential for infection by aerosols and in which the resulting disease may have serious or lethal consequences. Researchers in BSL-3 labs generally wear double gloves, respirators and disposable surgical scrubs and gowns, and work in biological safety cabinets in isolated, negative-pressure containment rooms. Some examples of BSL-3 organisms include *Mycobacterium tuberculosis, Bacillus anthracis, Brucella, Salmonella* typhi, *Francisella,* Plague bacilli, many arboviruses, Rickettsiae, Chlamydiae, Coccidioides, Histoplasma, HIV, etc.

BSL-4 organisms are easily transmitted, very high risk micro-organisms which cause life-threatening diseases for which there is no vaccine or therapy. Workers in BSL-4 labs work in impermeable positive pressure "space suits" with an external oxygen supply, and precautions, such as chemical showers must be taken before exiting the lab. Examples of BSL-4 organisms include Ebola virus, Marburg virus, Lassa fever virus Avian Influenza virus, etc.

The World Health Organization recommends that the health authorities of each country should make lists of the organisms and viruses in each biosafety level, as appropriate to local circumstances, so that suitable precautions may be applied.

No one list will suffice for all countries because circumstances will vary from one region to another. For example, if an organism is widespread in a community, there is no point in taking elaborate laboratory precautions to protect laboratory staff. Again there will be little need to protect the community if an infection is unlikely to spread because of the absence of vectors or as a result of good sanitation or other public health measures.

Experiment **1**

Orientation to a Virology Laboratory

Students must be aware of the basic procedures, instruments and equipments used in the virology Laboratory.

Filtration

Filtration technique has been used to separate viruses from bacteria and for many years as a criterion for the presence of a virus. If a filtrate proved infectious and no bacteria could be demonstrated, then a virus was presumed to be present. Filters of various porosities were manufactured and by passing a virus through series of filters having pores of known size, the approximate size of the virus was determined by noting which filter allowed the passage of the virus and which retained it. Filters are useful instrument for sterilization of certain thermo labile material like serum, trypsin solution, etc.

The filters remove bacteria either by mechanically withholding them from passing through the minute pores of filters or by absorption of bacteria to the filter because of the difference in their electrical charges.

The commonly used microbiological filters are:

1. **Berkefeld and Mandler filter** - These are made of diatomaceous earth and Berkefeld is graded into three porosity:
    a) V - (Viel) grade is coarse, used for preliminary filtration to remove some bacteria and large particles from a solution.
    b) N - (Normal) grade retains all bacteria while nearly all viruses will pass through.
    c) W - (Wenig) grade have very small pores and will retain all bacteria as well as some large viruses.

    Mandler filter is graded into preliminary, regular and fine grades.

2. Chamberland and Selas candle type filters - These are made of unglazed porcelain, moulded into a candle form chamberland is graded in porosities of Li-coarse grade to L13- the finest grade. Selas filters are graded from XF, XFF, No-10 and No-01, which are coarse grades to No-015, No-02 and No-03 which retain bacteria.
3. Seitz filter-These filters are asbestos pads manufactured in two grades - K, which is coarse, and EK, which retains bacteria. These pads are held in a metal holder and are discarded after being used once to eliminate cleaning. Sterilization of asbestos pad filter is done by autoclaving the pad assembled in its receptacle for 30 minutes at 121°C.
4. Sintered glass filter-These are made of fused porous glass. They are graded into specially fine ("grade 5") and a coarser ("grade 3") layer and is known as the 375" type. These filters are attached to the filtering apparatus in same way as Seitz filter.
5. Membrane filter-These are made of cellulose membrane or cellulose derivatives. They are manufactured in a variety of porosities. Those used in the virology are - coarse with the pore diameter 3μ to 0.75 μ medium 0.75 μ to 0.5 μ dense 0.5 μ to 0.2 μ and very dense below 0.2 μ.

Preparation of filters for use

Before a filter is used, it must be clean, sterile and free from leaks. New filter of the Berkefeld or Mandler type should be washed free of dust by passing distilled water through them from the outside to the inside of the filter and then reversing the flow.

Sterilization of filter of the moulded candle type is usually accomplished by autoclaving for 15 minutes at 121°C after which they are gradually cooled and allowed to dry.

Technique of filtration

The ideal condition of virus filtration is to remove bacteria but to allow the passage of all of the virus present in the solution.

The efficiency of filtration is dependent upon the following factors:

1. Size of virus to be passed
2. Amount of virus present.

3. Diameter of the pores of the filter.
4. Electrical charge of filter.
5. Electrical charge of the virus.
6. Amount of negative or positive pressure applied.
7. Viscosity and pH of the solution.
8. Duration of the filtering operation.

In this exercise, the working of seitz filter will be demonstrated to the student. The principle of working of other types of filters should also be explained by the instructor.

Materials

Seitz filter assembly, vacuum and pressure pump and the liquid for filtration.

Procedure

1. Connect the vacuum and pressure pump with the side nozzle of a safety device, which in its turn is connected to the Erlenmeyer flask of the filter assembly.
2. Pour liquid in the funnel of the filter and let the vacuum and pressure pump function. By means of negative pressure, the liquid will pass through the asbestos filter pad into the empty flask which will be bacteria free.

Successful filtration is to a great extent dependent upon knowledge of the porosities of the various filters and of the virus to be filtered. Obviously, a filter must be chosen which has pores larger than virus to be passed into the filtrate. On the other hand, the filter pores must be small enough to withhold bacteria, which may be present.

Glasswares and equipments for tissue culture work

Various types of material are used in cell culture as described below:

Glass Ware

The material must commonly used for growing cells is glass since it is readily available and is cheap and can be used repeatedly. All the glass wares used in cell culture should be of neutral type and the borosilicate glass is highly suitable for cultivating cells. The new glass wares may give a poor growth of cells even after careful washing but start giving satisfactory results, when used and once or twice. No satisfactory explanation is available but it is assumed that residual toxic ions inhibit the growth of cells at first time but are sufficiently removed afterwards to permit a good growth.

The following are the glass wares with their specification which are generally used in cell culture work:

Milk dilution Bottles (160 ml capacity)

This is used for growing monolayer cell culture is which stock virus is prepared. It is also suitable for plaque assay of viruses. The cell culture media may be also kept in them so that at one time one bottle is taken and the whole medium is consumed. 10 ml cell suspension is put in it.

Roux culture Bottles (1000 ml capacity)

It is suitable when virus production on large scale is desired. 100 ml cell suspension is put in these bottles.

Culture tube without rim (15 x 150 mm)

They are used for growing the cell culture either on their surfaces or on the cover slip inserted in them 1 ml or 2 ml cell suspension is added in them.

Leighton tubes

These are tubes as item no 3 except that a flat surface is made at inner side of the closed end of the tube so that coverslip is put in that flat area. It is quite convenient since the full cover slip may be accomodated.

Culture tubes, Round bottom with Screw cap and Rubber liner (15 x 155 mm)

It is used to grow the monolayer culture and requires 1 ml cell suspension.

Petridish culture (50 mm diameter)

It is suitable for growing monolayer culture and is of much use when doing plaque assay of the virus.

Trypsinizing flask

It is a special flask with corrugated wall and a spout and is suitable for separating the cells from tissue under the influence of enzyme trypsin.

In addition, several other types of glasswares like conical flask, beakers, pipettes, etc. are required. They are available in different capacities and the catalogue of corning should consulted for their specifications.

Plastic vessels

Polystyrene vessels and other items are now gaining wide use in cell culture and have been found highly suitable. They are suitably treated for cell culture growth and are presterilized so that they can be directly brought in use in the laboratory, this saves much of the time and investment in washing and preparation of glass ware in the laboratory.

Stoppers for culture vessels

Rubber stoppers are used for various culture vessels, such as tubes flasks, bottles, etc. They should be made from high quality rubber (i.e. silicon rubber) since the toxic substances released by inferior quality rubber are harmful to the cells as luckily to be spoiled in subsequent autoclaving they are available in different numbers like 1, 2, 3, etc. which fit into the mouth of glassware's of corresponding dimensions.

Rubber tubing

The same considerations as described for rubber stoppers apply to rubber tubing also silicon rubber tubing is highly satisfactory.

Equipments

The equipments used should be of a good quality. The following equipments are required in virus laboratory like deepfreeze, refrigerator, refrigerated centrifuge, lyophilizer, hot air oven, autoclave, water bath, incubator, magnetic stirrer with teflon coated magnetic bar, filters, vacuums pump, florescent microscope, inverted microscope, instrument sterilizer, laminar flow cabinets and ultra-violet lamp.

Appliances

Scissors, curved and straight, scalpels, forceps, curved and straight, aprons, face masks, hand gloves.

Washing Procedures (Washing of new glass wares)

1. New glass ware contains toxic products derived from manufacturing producer and packing they should be washed carefully.
2. Autoclave at 15 lb pressure for 50 min to 1 hrs.
3. Wash several times with tap water.
4. Immerse in a 4% solution of hydrochloric acid in water over night.
5. Rinse in tap water.
6. Immerse in detergent solution (soap powder or teepol) over night.
7. Scrub mechanically.
8. Rinse in tap water several times. To remove the detergent solution.
9. Rinse thrice in metal distilled water.
10. Rinse thrice in triple glass distilled water.

Washing of used glass wares

1. Scrub the glass wares with 10 per cent soap solution.
2. Wash thoroughly with tap water.
3. Rinse in 0.05 per cent HCI.
4. Wash thoroughly with tap water.
5. Rinse thrice in metal distilled water.
6. Rinse thrice with triple glass distilled water.

Washing of Rubber corks (Bungs)

The above mentioned procedure is followed for those which are in use. The new rubber corks received from the firm are subjected to the following treatment after autoclaving at 15 lbs pressure for 30 minutes:

1. Boil for 15 minutes in 20 per cent sodium bicarbonate or sodium hydroxide solution.
2. Rinse in hot tap water
3. Boil for 15 minutes in 20 per cent hydrochloride acid solution.
4. Rinse in hot tap water.
5. Rinse thrice with metal distilled water followed by triple glass distilled water.

Washing of filters

It is ideal that seitz filter pads should be washed free of alkali and asbestos fibers by passing considerable amount of sterile glass distilled water.

Sintered glass filters should be cleaned with strong acids after use. Concentrated sulphuric acid to which few crystals of sodium nitrate and sodium chlorate have been added is passed through the filter. After this, filter should be rinsed with a large volume of glass distilled water.

Pipettes

1. Wash in tap water
2. Boil in appropriate detergent solution for 10 min.
3. Wash in continuous flow pipette washed for 4 h.
4. Rinse in de-ionized water

Syringes

1. Pour off disinfectant and rinse in tap water.
2. Boil in appropriate detergent for 10 min.
3. Rinse in tap water
4. Boil in deionized water.

Siliconed glass wares

1. Remove the silicone grease from the glassware with benzene.
2. Place the glass ware in grease remover for a few hours.

Grease remover

50% potassium hydroxide	50 ml
Methanol	850 ml

Do further washing in the normal ways as described for used glasswares.

Washing of metallic appliances

All the appliances, such as scalpels, scissors, forceps, etc. may be boiled in 10% soap solution and then washed as described for glass wares.

Drying and preparation of glasswares and apparatus

All the materials after washing should be immediately dried in a hot air oven at 60-70°C. The tubes, flasks, beakers, etc. should be kept inverted so that water comes out quickly and drying is completed soon.

After drying, the mouths of the vessels are plugged with cotton wool wrapped in muslin cloth and then wrapped with aluminium foil and sent for sterilization.

Sterilization

The purpose of sterilization is to destroy all the living organisms, which could be the source of contamination. Two methods are used for sterilization of glass wares and apparatus.

Dry Heat

Sterilization by dry heat is done in a hot air oven, it is a method of choice for all glassware's and apparatus which do not contain any material which could be destroyed the sterilization is done at 160°C for 60 min or at 180 for 30 min.

High pressure steam

High pressure steam sterilization is done in the autoclave. All the apparatus which cannot be sterilized by dry heat are sterilized in the autoclave, the sterilization should be done at 15 lb/in^2 pressure for 20-30 min.

Media and Reagent

The medium is the most important factor in culturing the cells in vitro. The function of the medium is to provide physical conditions, such as pH, O_2, CO_2, osmotic pressure, and nutrition to the cells in the form of chemical substances, such as amino acids, carbohydrates and vitamins. The water used in the preparation of the medium for dissolving these ingredients should be very pare, preferably triple glass distilled. An ordinary medium may contain lactalbumin hydrolysate, yeast extract and serum in a balanced salt solution. The serum is one of the most important growth promoting substances and is essential for the satisfactory growth of the cells. The foetal calf serum has been found to be quite satisfactory and essential for cell lines for primary cell cultures, the serum collected from a young calf may serve the purpose. For cell lines chemically defined media which contain all the required salt, amino acids, vitamins, etc. are used along with the foetal calf serum.

Distilled water

For cell culture work double or triple glass distilled water, should be used. It is better to use metal distilled water for putting into the glass distillation apparatus so that calcium and other salts do not logg the distillation apparatus readily. It is advisable to add a few crystals of potassium permanganate to tap water before commencing distillation so that they may oxidize the steam volatile organic compounds which might otherwise be carried over into the distillate.

Check the purity of the distilled water by the conductivity test, it should have conductivity below 1 PPM of sodium chloride.

Demineralised or de ionized water prepared in deionize units whose inner surface is made of good quality stainless steel may also be used.

❑❑❑

Experiment 2

Collection, Preservation, Transport of Samples and their Processing in Virology Laboratory

On the face of an outbreak or a disease, collection of clinical specimens in proper preservative, their transportation to the laboratory under ideal conditions, and quick processing of the specimens in the laboratory to identify the causative agent are crucial to successful treatment and control of the disease.

Collection of specimens is done for three purposes:

1. Specimens for virus isolation.
2. Specimens for serological investigation.
3. Specimens for direct examination (rapid diagnosis).

The specimens for virus isolation are usually taken from the affected regions. Thus, throat swabs or nasal swabs are taken when the infection involves the upper respiratory tract, and sputum is taken from the lower respiratory tract infections. Scrapings are taken from the lesions of the skin and mucous membranes, and if vesicles are present at these sites, the vesicle fluid is also removed. Blood is withdrawn in the cases of rash. Signs referable to central nervous system (CNS) involvement indicate the collection of cerebrospinal fluid, but since such involvement may be due to one of the large number of viruses whose normal habitat is the alimentary tract, stools or rectal swab are also obtained. The latter may be required in addition from cases of infection with the more stable respiratory disease agents, such as certain adenoviruses and reoviruses.

In the case of serum, two serum samples, one at the beginning and another 1-2 weeks later, are taken to show the rise or fall of the antibody level. The following points should be remembered while selecting the specimens:

1. The titer of viruses is usually the highest at the affected sites and during the early stages of the disease.
2. In diseases where viremia is noticed, the maximum titer of the virus often coincides with peak pyrexia and may precede the onset of other clinical signs.
3. Secondary bacterial infection is a common sequel of virus diseases. As such, samples taken from the later stages of the disease or at postmortem are less likely to contain viable virus. The selection of specimens in relation to the disease has been shown in table.

Table Samples to be collected in different diseases

Disease	Sample	
	Live animal	Postmortem
Respiratory and ocular disease	Nasal and conjunctival swabs, blood, etc.	Tissues from selected areas of the affected organ and the associated lymph-nodes
Skin diseases and lesions of mucous membranes of mouth and genital tract	Scrapings of lesions, swabs from affected area and blood	Tissues from affected area and the associated lymph-nodes
Gastroenteritis	Faeces, blood	Intestinal contents
Systemic disease	Blood, nasal and urogenital swabs and faeces	Tissues from various organs including lymph-nodes, liver
Diseases of CNS	Blood, CSF, faeces, nasal and urogenital swabs	Tissues of selected areas of affected system and the associated lymph-nodes
Disease of urinary tract	Urogenital swab, urine and blood	Tissues of selected areas of affected system and the associated lymph-nodes
Abortion	Blood fromdam, vaginal mucous, Uterine discharge	Tissues from placenta , cotyledons, whole or affected organs of fetus, blood from fetal heart, intestinal contents

The term blood in table refers to the clotted sample for serology and the sample collected with anticoagulant for other tests; 5 to 20 ml of blood may be collected. Whenever possible, the clot should be removed before dispatch.

Specimens for direct examination are also collected as described for virus isolation but smears are aid for rapid testing using immunofluorescence or immunoenzyme techniques.

Method of collection Nasal swabs

The posterior nasal passages are most likely to contain viruses; hence posterior nasal swabs should be collected. The swab is prepared by twisting long stable cotton on to a stick. The stick and the cotton should be sterilized in a hot air oven. The swab is moistened with transport medium immediately before use, then it is introduced into the nostril and carefully pushed along with the floor in the nasal passage as far as possible. It is then gently rotated until it becomes generously coated with nasal secretion. The swab is then removed and it is placed into the bottle containing the transport medium, the extra stick is broken off, and the vial is capped.

Throat swabs

The swabs as used for nasal swabs may serve the purpose but the stick should be long. The tongue should be pressed on one side the swab moisted and the opposite posterior pharyngeal wall are rubbed around. The procedure is repeated on the other side, the swab is placed in a bottle, the extra stick is broken off, and the vial is capped.

Rectal swab

The type of the nasal or throat swab may suffice. The swab is inserted without moistening slowly through the anal sphincter into the rectum and rotated gently. Then, it is withdrawn and placed in the bottle containing the transport medium.

Faecal sample

It should be collected direct from the rectum of the animal and placed in a vial.

Cerebrospinal fluid

1. The site for cerebrospinal fluid withdrawal is in the lumbosacral foramen observed by digital manipulation from the sacrum posteriorly and the last lumbar vertebra anteriorly.
2. Shave the site and wash with soap and water.
3. Apply 70% alcohol.
4. Collect the cerebrospinal fluid with the help of 18 gauge 2 in needle and syringe and transfer it to a tube.

Oesophagopharyngeal fluid (OP fluid)

Some of the viruses localize in the pharyngeal region and it is advantageous to collect the pharyngeal scrapings. This is done using a probang cup. The probang cup is inserted into the mouth upto the pharyngeal region and moved up and down so as to collect scrapings of the pharyngeal wall and fluid. It should be withdrawn slowly and the contents placed in the transport medium.

Vesicle fluid

With the help of a 1-ml syringe fitted with a fine needle the vesicle fluid is collected by slowly inserting the needle and simultaneously withdrawing the plunger. The fluid is placed in a small volume (1-ml) of transport medium.

Lesion scrapings

A sterile scalpel and a forceps are used to collect the skin scrapings. The epithelial covering of the vesicle is collected with the help of the forceps and placed in the transport medium.

Blood

Blood is collected with a syringe containing heparin (20 III heparin/ml blood).

Serum

Blood is collected in a tube and is kept at 4°C to allow the formation of a clot. When the clot retracts, it is centrifuged at 3000 rpm for 15 min and the supernatant serum collected.

Post mortem materials

These are collected either for virus isolation or for pathological examination or for direct demonstration of viral antigen in tissues. For virus isolation, they are collected in 50% buffered glycerine and for pathological examination in buffered formalin saline containing 10% formalin.

Table - Collections of materials of some important animal diseases

Disease	Materials to be collected
Bovine Ephemeral fever	Heparinized citrated or defibrinated blood for transmission test; paired sera for SN test.
Malignant catarrhal fever	Citrated or defibrinated blood; mucous membrane smears (air-dried, sent in ice box), lymph-nodes of head and neck, pieces of liver and/or spleen in buffered glycerine, pieces of brain, liver spleen, kidney, adrenals, nasal mucosa in 10% formal saline.
Rinderpest	Defibrinated or citrated blood; pieces of lymph-node, spleen in 50% glycerine salines; intestinal lesions in 10% formalin
Mucosal diseases virus diarrhoea	Defibrinated or citrated blood; Lesions from mouth, gut, peyer's patches; lymph-nodes, spleen, liver and kidney in 50% glycerine saline
Foot and mouth disease	Vesicular fluid in transport medium; Vesicular epithelium from dorsum of tongue, gum, dental pad in 50% buffered glycerine
Infectious bovine rhinotracheitis/infectious vulvovaginitis	Nasal and conjunctival swabs in transport media; swabs from genital tract in transport media; paired serum samples for serum neutralization test. Affected trachea and turbinate bones, lung, kidney in 10% formalin
Bovine enterovirus	Aborted fetal contents heart, liver, lung
Cowpox, Buffalo pox	Skin scrapings and vesicular fluid in transport media
Influenza and parainfluenza	Nasal swabs in transport medium; paired sera samples.
Blue tongue	Nasal swabs, tongue epithelium in transport medium; citrated blood and paired sera samples

Louping ill	Citrated blood, paired sera samples, brain in 50% glycerine saline
Visna and Maedi	Citrated blood, CSF and saliva in transport medium, brain, lungs and spleen in 50% glycerine saline
Duck virus hepatitis	Blood, liver in buffered glycerine
Infectious Bronchitis	Bursa, kidney in buffered glycerine
African Horse Sickness	Citrated blood, paired sera samples, spleen, lymph-nodes and brain on ice

Transportation of Clinical Specimens

The viability of viruses is adversely affected by exposure to temperature, extremes of pH, most common disinfectants, light, irradiation, and desiccation. It is, therefore, necessary to protect the sample during the interval between its collection and processing. Specimens taken in small amounts viz., swabs and skin scrapings are most likely to be affected by ambient conditions and should be placed in a suitable medium.

The two common virus transport media used are: (1) 50% glycerine phosphate buffer saline, and (2) hank's balanced salt solution (HBSS) containing 0.5% bovine serum albumin and antibiotics.

Transport medium

Bovine serum albumin	5g
Penicillin	10 lakh units
Streptomycin	1 g
Mycostatin	25000 units
BSS	1000 ml

As soon as the specimen is collected, it should be maintained at an optimum pH (7.2-7.4) and should be transported on ice, if virus isolation is to be attempted. The specimens for pathological examination and fixed in formal saline can be transported without any preservative. The specimens should usually not be frozen because freezing and thawing may destroy the infectivity as well as lower the virus content. Hence, it would be advisable to store such specimens at 4°C and try to process them within 24 hrs.

Sera samples and blood may be transported at room temperature and stored at 4°C in the laboratory.

Containers

Each container should consist of a vial, made up of strong neutral glass, and have a screw top of cap complete with a rubber liner or washer so that no leakage occurs. After putting the material in the bottle/vial with the medium, and closing of the top, the outside of the vial should be disinfected either with 4% sodium carbonate or with 0.2% citric acid solution. The screw cap should be sealed by winding around with an adhesive tape. Another piece of adhesive tape should be put on the vial on which are recorded the identification particulars of the sample.

The vial then should be wrapped in adsorbent cotton wool/lint/ corrugated paper and put into a metal container. The metal container, in turn, should have a screw top complete with a rubber washer or liner so as to be leak proof. The metal container should then be placed in a strong outer carton of wood or reinforced cardboard and securely wrapped.

The details or the origin/source of the sample and its identification particulars for reference should be given. As much information as possible to gather should be given. One copy of the information pertaining to the sample must be sent with the sample and another copy sent separately to the laboratory.

Dispatch of sample

The parcel should preferably be dispatched immediately through a courier, air flight, or otherwise posted by mail, according to exigencies and facilities available. At the same time intimation may be sent to the concerned laboratory by cable/letter about the dispatch of the sample.

Labelling of parcels containing sample

The samples sent by air flight/post in the form of a parcel must bear a label marked as follows:

- Do not open infective biological material fragile with care, perishable biologicals.

- Parcels to/from overseas countries should be added with "No commercial value". The address of the laboratory to which it is sent should be written/printed correctly and legibly along with the stander's address.

Preparation of Clinical Specimens Swabs

An identical procedure is used for the preparation of nasal throat, rectal, and veside swabs. The swab is macerated well in the transport medium itself used for collection. The resulting suspension is transferred to a centrifuge tube and centrifuged at 3000-5000 rpm for 20 min. The supernatant is collected and inoculated into the susceptible host and stored at freezing temperature.

Feces

10% suspension of the faecal materials made using the transport medium with a screw capped bottle coarse glass beads are added and shaken vigorously. The suspension is poured into centrifuge tubes and centrifuged at 10 rpm for 20 min at 4°C in a refrigerated centrifuge. If this speed is not possible because of the absence of such a centrifuge, it is centrifuged at 3000-5000 rpm for 20 min. The upper two-thirds of the supernatant fluid is removed for inoculation and stored at 20°C.

Vesicle fluid

It is centrifuged as described in swabs and inoculated using the supernatant.

Lesion scrapings

Scraping, such as vesicle crusts, pock lesions, and tongue epithelium removed from the buffered glycerine, put in a mortar and washed several times with PBS. Then using coarse washed sand, it is triturated thoroughly and a 10% suspension made in BSS. It is centrifuged at 3000 rpm for 20 min and the supernatant collected.

Postmortem material Process as described for lesion scrapings

Preparation of washed sand

1. Add about five volumes of 1 N HCI to one volume of white sand, and soak overnight at room temperature.

2. Wash in running tap water until the effluent is no longer acid.
3. Wash at least ten times in de ionized water, adding ten volumes of water and stirring well at each stage.
4. After the last washing, drain the sand completely and tip on to several thickness of filter paper.
5. Cover and dry at 180°C-200°C.
6. Sterilize in a hot-air oven (160°C for 1 hr).

□□□

Experiment 3

Isolation of Viruses

From clinical specimen, virus can be isolated by inoculating into any of the hosts mentioned below depending upon the susceptibility and practical availability.

A) In laboratory animals or poultry

Animal inoculation was the first method of virus cultivation and for many years was the only means of virus propagation. This method is not convenient and is also more expensive than embryo method. Besides serving to propagate the virus, the inoculation of various animal host is important in the identification of an unknown virus.

To confirm the infectious nature of a disease, it may be necessary to reproduce the clinical illness in another member of the same species; either by placing healthy susceptible animals in direct contact with those showing symptoms of infection or by inoculating groups of healthy and immune (vaccinated) animals by a suitable route with a material obtained by a sick animal. If the later procedure is adopted, it is necessary to insure that the material capable of transmitting the disease does not contain other micro-organisms (example bacteria) which produce a concurrent infection and complicate the clinical picture. To insure that the inoculum is bacteriological sterile the material must be filtered or treated with antibiotics.

In medical virology, monkeys are frequently used for inoculation since it is possible to reproduce in these species many human diseases which show similar clinical symptoms and comparable development.

In veterinary medicine, the same species or at least those closely related to the host animal should be used and in diseases, such as swine fever, which show a high degree of host specificity the use of same species may be obligatory.

On the other hand many viruses including some members of the togavirus group can be grown successfully and will produce clinical disease in a wide variety of laboratory animals, such as dogs, cats, mice, rats, guinea pig, rabbits and hamsters as well as producing abnormalities of developing chicken embryo and a variety of cell culture.

Animal inoculation is used in distinguishing between viruses, which produce similar lesion, such as foot and mouth disease and vesicular stomatitis of cattle. In such cases calves and horses are inoculated. Calves are susceptible to both viruses while horses are insusceptible to foot and mouth disease virus but readily contact vesicular stomatitis.

The natural host is still being used for studies of pathogenesis, immunology, vaccine trials, diagnosis and chemotherapy.

Rabies diagnosis in some case must be made by the inoculation of the laboratory animals because Negri bodies cannot always be demonstrated in the brain of the infected animal.

Viruses which produce encephalitis are usually inoculated intracerebrally, the pox viruses intradermally, intranasally and those of the respiratory group and example of other types of inoculation include inoculation into the scarified cornea of a rabbit, scarified epithelium of the mouth and tongue of calves or the foot pad of the guinea pig.

In poultry, inoculation of live virus vaccine is made into the feathered follicles on the leg, the web of the wing, or in the case of laryngo tracheitis vaccine, into the cloacal bursa.

The experimental animals must be healthy, before they are used and that they be properly cared for during the course of the experiment. Not only are laboratory animals prone to a wide variety of bacterial, viral and parasitic diseases, which may complicate the result of a particular experiment; but they are also liable to harbor various latent or subclinical infections, which may be activated under the stress of a particular experiment. These difficulties are largely overcome if specific pathogen free stock, or gnotobiotic facilities are available before and during an experiment the operator should personally examine the animals once or preferably, twice daily for the detection of the signs of the disease or other abnormalities. Whereever possible, rectal temperatures should be taken and recorded daily by means of a blunt clinical thermometer.

The experiment animals are used for virus isolation, to study pathogenecity and host immune reactions, develop viral vaccines and to raise monoclonal or polyclonal antibodies.

1. Virus isolation - For diagnostic purposes the experimental animals are still used for example mice in rabies and louping ill disease diagnosis.

2. To study pathogenicity and host immune reactions- This is studied in homologous host example pig in swine fever. The cost of using the homologous host is very high and therefore, inbred experimental animals are used instead of homologous host. Example inbred mice used in African swine fever. The laboratory animals used as models are:

   a) Rabbit - the rabbits were used by the Pasteur to adopt street virus of rabies. In malignant catarrhal fever virus, these animals react in the similar manner as the cattle.

   b) Guinea pig - guinea pigs react to foot and mouth disease virus when inoculated intradermaly in the footpad. Primary vesical is formed on the footpad and secondary vesicals appear in the mouth following viraemia.

   c) Ferrets - ferrets are used in the study of pathogenesis of distemer virus.

   Other laboratory animals are also used in virus study or in the preparation of antisera against different viruses.

3. To test and develop viral vaccines - Mice, guinea pig, rabbits are used for attenuation of virus strains as well as for testing vaccines. Foot and mouth disease virus vaccine is initially tested in guinea pigs and finally in cattle and pigs.

4. To raise monoclonal or polyclonal antibodies- Various routes are employed to inoculate experimental animals with virus infected material. The usual routes are intracerebral, intranasal, intradermal, intramuscular, intravenous and subcutaneous, the route of inoculation largely depends upon the nature of virus; its possible affinity for the tissue, age and species of experimental animal.

Preparation of inoculum

The material used for animal inoculation may consist of filtered or unfiltered suspensions of organs or exudates. If the materials are unfiltered, it is important to add antibacterial substance, such as penicillin and streptomycin, to prevent contaminating or associated bacterial agent from becoming established. This is especially important in intracerebral inoculation, some bacteria which are ordinarily considered non pathogenic may cause infection, when directly introduced into the brain tissue of the living animal.

A general procedure for the Preparation of inoculum is as follows:

1. The infected tissue or exudate is removed from the animal with sterile instrument and placed in a sterile container.
2. The tissue is cut into small pieces and placed in a sterile mortar.
3. An abrasive, such as sterile alundum (90 mesh) is sprinkled over the tissue which is ground to a paste and then suspended in tryptose phosphate broth or other buffered liquid to make a 10-12% suspension.
4. Centrifugation at 3000 rpm for 3-5 minutes will clarify the material so that the supernatant can be used in a syringe for injection.
5. After centrifugation the supernatant fluid is transferred to another tube and the antibiotics are added.
6. A period of 15-30 minutes incubation at room temperature is allowed before the mixture is injected. However, if the material is collected relatively free of contamination, it can be inoculated immediately into animals and chicken embryos.

Inoculation technique

The usual routes of commonly employed for the inoculation of the viruses into experimental animals are - intravenous, intramuscular, subcutaneous, intradermal, intraperitoneal, intracerebral and Intranasal. In addition, other routes of inoculation viz. intraplantar, intradermolingual, corneal, scarification, cheek pouch and per oral may also be employed in certain specialized cases.

The sizes of the hypodermic needles are expressed as s.w.g. x inches. The abbreviation s.w.g. denotes standard wire gauge, which is the diameter of the needle. The larger is the s.w.g. number the smaller will be the needle diameter, thus 26 s.w.g. needle is a very fine one as compared with a 18 s.w.g needle. The length of the needle from the mount to the point is given in inches.

Route of Inoculation Intravenous

Monkey, rabbits, mice and rats may be inoculated by this route. Inoculation into an ear vein may be done with a fine needle, otherwise a vein in the leg should be used for inoculation. In monkey femoral vein is used for inoculation.

1. For inoculation into rabbits, the ear should be warmed by applying warm water to dilute the vein.
2. The injection site should be cleaned with alcohol.
3. When the alcohol dries up, a one inch 26 s.w.g needle is inserted into the marginal vein and when it is felt that the needle is inside the vein, the plunger is slightly withdrawn until a little blood is withdrawn. This will ensure that needle is in the correct position.
4. Then, the inoculum is injected slowly. The average dose is 0.5 ml but upto 2.5 ml may be injected.

Mice and rats may be injected into the caudal vein

1. The tail should be immersed in warm water (55°C) to dilate the caudal vein.
2. Inoculation is done with a 1 inch 26 s.w.g needle.
3. Volume of 0.5 ml in rats and 0.2 ml in mice is injected.

In chick, inoculation is done into the humoral vein

1. One assistant should hold the bird in supine-position with the wing well-spread.
2. Enough feather are plucked to expose the vein, where it passes along the inner side of the wing in the humoral region.
3. Inoculation is done with a 1 inch 26 s.w.g needle

4. The needle is inserted into the vein and the proper placing is ascertained by moving the needle to and fro and slightly withdrawing the plunger to see if some blood is withdrawn.
5. After which the inoculum is injected upto 5 ml volume may be injected.

Intramuscular

It is very simple inoculation for which a suitable muscle may be used and usually thigh muscle is selected. In rodents, inoculation is done into the gastrocnemius muscle with a 0.5-inch (1.27-cm) inch 26 s.w.g needle. The needle is inserted about 2-3 mm into the flesh part and 0.05 ml is gently inoculated. In rabbits 1 ml in one leg may be inoculated.

Subcutaneous

Any area of the animal where the skin is loose may be used. In rabbits and mice, injection may be between the shoulders. A fold of skin should be punched between the under finger and the thumb and injection made through the fold. In large animals, the loose skin along the flank may be used.

Intradermal

Any suitable site may be chosen. The hair is removed to wash the site with water. The injection is made by inserting the needle horizontally at an angle so that the needle does not penetrate deep makes the injection.

Intraperitoneal

All the laboratory animals are suitable for this inoculation, the inoculation is made to one side of the midline of the lower abdomen. As the needle is withdrawn, the skin around it should be gently pinched together and held for a few seconds to prevent the inoculum from leaking back. For mice, the animal is held horizontally, the ventral surface uppermost and the needle is inserted (1 inch 23 s.w.g.) through the abdominal wall about 5 mm lateral to the mid line, at an angle of about 30° from the horizontal. The needle is inserted 1 cm. deep to avoid puncturing of the viscera. A volume of 0.5 to 2 ml is usually injected although upto 5 ml may be inoculated.

Intracerebral

In a suckling mouse, no assistance is required. The mouse is held firmly on the bench with the left hand in the sitting position of the mouse (dorsal surface uppermost) a % inch 26 s.w.g. needle is inserted vertically through the left cranial wall at a point equidistant from the anterior margin of the ear, the posterior angle of the eye and the cranial mid line. The needle is inserted to about 2 mm, 0.01 ml is inoculated and the needle withdrawn.

In an adult mouse and other animals, anesthesia is required. In an adult mouse, the animal is anaesthetized with ether and placed on the bench, the remaining procedure is the same as described, above for a suckling mouse. The needle is inserted about 2 to 3 mm, 0.03 ml is inoculated and the needle is withdrawn.

For rabbits and monkeys, drilling of a hole is required for inoculation to be done.

Intranasal

Mice and ferrets are usually employed for this route and inoculation is done with a 0.5 inch 23 s.w.g. needle which should have a blunt tip. The animal is anaesthetized, the animal is held keeping the head up, the needle is brought to the nostril and the required inoculum (0.05 ml in mice & 0.1 ml in ferrets) is dropped slowly.

Intraplanter

The route is employed for such disease as mousepox and foot and mouth disease in which case the planter pad (foot pad) is inoculated. For foot and mouth disease, guinea pigs are employed. A 1.5 inch 22 s.w.g. needle, whose tip has been made slightly blunt by a little grinding is used. The assistant should hold the guinea pig. The toes are held with the left hand by keeping them pressed with the thumb and the needle is inserted with the right hand. Several tunnels are made intradermally and inoculum injected. The volume of inoculation is 0.1 ml in each pad. It is also called interadermal pad inoculation.

Intradermolingual

This route is specially used for inoculating apthovirus (foot and mouth disease virus) in cattle. No sterilization of the inoculation area is done. The tongue of the animal is withdrawn and held tightly by taking the tip of the touque in the grip by the assistant. A 1/ 1/2 inches 26 s.w.g. needle is inserted intradermally into the tongue by keeping the needle horizontal to the tongue surface and making tunnels. It starts from the inner side of the tongue making several tunnels and then coming towards the tip about five lines of the tunnels with five tunnels in each line are made.

Corneal scarification

This route is employed in rabbit. No sterilization of the inoculation area is required. The animal is anaesthetized with ether and placed on its side. One drop of inoculum is placed on the corneal surface and gently scarified with the scalpel blade.

Cheek pouch

Hamsters are inoculated by this route. No sterilization of the inoculation is done. The animal is anaesthetized with ether and its mouth open using the left thumb and the index finger the cheek pouch is held, the animal leg suspended and the mucous membrane of the cheek pouch is exposed for inoculation. A ½ inch, 26 s.w.g. needle is introduced into the pouch tissue as superficially as possible and slowly 0.1 ml inoculated. This route is employed for studying the oncogenic viruses for their ability to produce tumors in hamsters.

Per oral

This route is employed in a few circumstances. The usual procedure is to hold the head high, to open the mouth, and to drop the inoculum into the posterior part of the buckle cavity and to keep the head high for some time and allow the animal to swallow the content.

Bleeding techniques

The experimental animal may be bled either by vein puncture or by cardiac puncture. The vein puncture is preferred, when small volume of blood are to be recovered.

Monkey

Bleeding is done from the femoral vein using a syringe with a 1½ inch 21 s.w.g needle attached. The animal should be anaesthetized before bleeding.

Rabbit

For routine purpose where a small volume of blood is required, bleeding may be done from the marginal ear vein without any anesthetic. To distant the vein and make it clearly visible, the area is swabbed with xylene or alcohol.

If a larger volume of blood is required, bleeding is done from the heart. The animal is placed in supine position and the position of the heart is located by palpating with finger. This may be done by keeping the fingers slightly over the left thoracic wall. The needle is inserted through the chest wall towards the heart and as soon as the needle touches the heart, the heartbeat is felt. The needle is pushed inside the heart in one stroke and the plunger is slightly withdrawn so that blood entire the syringe freely. The required volume of blood is withdrawn and the needle is removed.

Rat, mouse, hamster

For a small volume, the bleeding may be done from the retro ocular plexus of veins of the eye. A pasture pipette is specially prepared for this purpose. A pasture pipette is taken and the tip is cut with a glass cutting foil at a place so that the diameter of the tip is about 1ml. The tip is ground to make it blunt so that it may not cause any injury. The assistant will hold the animal keeping the dorsal surface uppermost. The eyelids are open with the left thumb and index finger and the tip of the pasture pipette is placed with the right hand in the orbital cavity without damaging the eye. This will result in bulging of eye to one side. The pipette is pushed further so that its tip touches the reto-ocular plexus and the pasture pipette is rotated and then slightly the pressure of pipette is loosened to allow the blood to be sucked in by capillary action. After the blood is sucked in, the pasture pipette is withdrawn and the blood is transferred into a small tube.

When a large volume of blood is required, it is collected either from the heart or by sacrificing the animal.

Chicken

Blood is withdrawn from the humoral vein with a 1 inch 21 s.w.g. needle. The bird is placed in a supine position with the wing well spread. The feathers are plucked to expose the vein. The needle is inserted in the vein and its correct position is ascertained by withdrawing the plunger, when the blood will flow in the syringe. The required volume of blood is collected and the needle is withdrawn.

Cattle, sheep, goat

Blood is collected from the jugular vein. The hair is removed and the jugular vein is pressed with the left thumb so that the flow of blood is stopped and the vein becomes prominent. The needle is inserted and the blood will flow immediately with force, if needle is placed rightly. The desired volume of blood is collected and the needle is withdrawn. For bleeding large volumes of blood, bleeding canula may be used.

It may be an advantage to withdraw blood samples at regular intervals from experimental animals to detect the possible development of specific antibodies (e.g. Q fever) and to cull and carry out post-mortem examination of some animals during the course of the experiment. Clinical symptoms, the development of visible lesions, abnormal behaviour and all deaths, whatever the cause, should be carefully observed and recorded. At the termination of an experiment involving infectious material, all bedding utensils cages, carcasses and tissues should be removed, burned, sterilized or thoroughly cleaned by the most appropriate method. Animals infected experimentally must be held in separate isolation rooms and all persons handling infected animals, cages or other contaminated materials must pay strict attention to personal cleanliness.

Special care must be taken when performing inclusions, if the material is believed to contain virulent viruses or when specimens obtained from experimentally infected animals are being processed for further passage in animals or inoculated into eggs or cell cultures.

B) Embryonated chicken eggs

Embryonated chicken egg inoculations were first used in the 1911 with propagation of virus by Roux and Marfey. In 1931, Woodruff and Goodpasture cultivated fowl poxvirus on the chorioallantoic membrane. Burnet used chicken embryo for cultivation of viruses very extensively. Since that time and until mid-1950 almost all research and testing with viruses depended on animal or embryonated eggs for source of living tissue. Later on there were replaced gradually by tissue culture which is now most commonly used for propagation of viruses. The embryonating egg is nevertheless still a convenient and easily manipulated source of living tissue for propagation and testing of virus.

The use of fertile hen's egg in diagnostic virology has a number of advantages:

1. Readily available, cheap and easily maintained.
2. Sheltered from the natural diseases often observed in laboratory animals and are relatively free from bacterial and many latent virus infections.
3. Easily manipulated under sterile conditions.
4. Generally free from natural factors of defense, specific or non-specific, that some time intervene and prevent passage in adult animals.
5. Sensitive to some virus that are harmless to the adult birds.
6. Easily identified and labeled with the details of the date, nature of the virus and the experimental procedure.

Facilities and Equipments

Small commercial egg incubators which are equipped to supply balance of heat, humidity and air circulation are most ideal. Generally incubation of embryonating egg should occur under following condition:

Temperature 37.5°C

Humidity 62%

Forced air circulation to ensure abalanced temperature and automatic turning trays to rotate the eggs during incubation.

Candling area and Equipments

A candling room should be dark, adequately ventilation and have 4 to 5 feet space to accommodate person during candling. If not available construct divides setting of a part of lab bench in corner or install black photographic curtain at height suspended from wall mounted.

Equipment needed are suitable light source apparatus to make small holes in shell of eggs. Candling lamps are available. An egg punch or drill commercially available is used in making shell pores. If this is unavailable, the sterile needle or rubber cork with an all-pin can be used.

Inoculation Area Equipments

Ideal inoculation area is a small room, which need not exceed 5 feet length. It should have lab lamp space and an area for equipment. It should preferably have a laminar flow benches fitted with ultraviolet lighting. To attain a clean room atmosphere, where facilities permit several inoculation rooms should be constructed. It is performed that each type of virus be handled in isolation. This avoid danger of contaminating the strain with each other. Under no circumstances, inoculation or harvesting of one virus should be done in a room where other have been handled recently unless cleaning of surface of entire room has been done.

Egg Supply

Certain information about egg supplying flock should be a part of equipment data. Following points should be recorded for all eggs used - Flock immunization history:

a) Type of vaccine used, date of manufacture, dose and route of administration.

b) Tests results on evaluation

c) *Production records* - It is essential to purchase egg from a single producer who can supply the necessary information, preferably have your own hatchery supply the eggs. The present international standards as laid down by WHO, OIE and EDA of various countries emphasize that specific pathogen free (SPF) embryonated eggs be used for propagation of virus either for research or production.

Anatomy of Embryonated Egg

The term "embryonated egg" identifies any eggs in which an embryo is developing. It is common to refer to fertile egg which have been incubated as being 3,5,10 days, etc. This does not refer to the time that has been exposed since the egg was laid but to the time that it has been incubated. Although certain early primitive developmental stages occur of fertilization and while the shell wall forms around egg contents. This development does not continues after bird lay eggs. Subsequently, when incubated artificially further development occurs. This potential does not lost so long as eggs are not subject to extreme of temperature, it is this characteristic of suspended development which make it possible for avian to production their natural habitat.

Shell and Shell Membrane

With sharp pointed forceps gently pick away shell of egg; a thin white membrane is seen, known as shell membrane. Outermost hard calcareous whitish covering of egg is egg shell. The shell function as an exchange system across its surface. Gaseous and liquid molecule passes in both directions. This is why the egg are incubated in presence of humidity and adequate circulation. If an egg is incubated in an atmosphere too low in humidity, it will use its moisture. The content will be dehydrated and the death of the embryo will result. Same is true for circulation. If embryonated eggs are tightly packed for too long period under incubator, the impairment of circulation will result in embryo death.

Air Space

All normal eggs have a rounded end and opposite to this is the end formed by more acute angle of shell that is pointed end under the shell and shell membrane of the blunt rounded end its an empty space. The egg contents are prevented from entering this area by layering of several membranes, which act as a barrier. The space is called air shell or air space. It functions both in respiration and pressure adjustment.

Isolation of viruses in laboratory animals or poultry or embryonated chicken eggs

Chorio allantoic sac/ membrane (CAM)

Attached to developing embryo and originating hindgut, is a sac whose function is to remove wastes. As the embryo increases in size the sac also enlarges until it surrounds the embryo much like a double layered umbrella. Membrane which forms the sac is usually called chorio allantoic membrane together with the content of sac is designated as CAS or allantoic cavity. The fluid content in sac is known as allantoic fluid. It is necessary to differentiate between CAM inoculation, when intend is to place the virus on/in membrane CAS or AF inoculation where intend is to place the virus in the allantoic fluid, allantoic cavity formed by CAM.

Yolk Sac and Yolk

Not only there is a CAS extending from developing embryo but structure called the yolk sac completely surround the yolk sac contents of the egg through its membrane and blood vessels, metabolites of yolk are transferred to embryos. As the embryo matures contents of yolk sac noticeably diminishes until the sac is approximately 1 cm. in diameter about three days before embryo hatch. At this state the embryo has attained such size that it nearly fills the egg and except for small opening in its abdomen from which yolk is produced the embryo is perfectly formed.

In the final days remaining to hatching time, the opening of abdomen fills slowly and the contents will be absorbed in the digestive system of embryo.

Amniotic Sac

This vary with membrane system is most easily seen in embryo of 4 to 9 days. It appears as translucent clear liquid field stretched over developing embryo. Infact, it is completely surrounding embryo except for areas, where chorio allantoic sac and yolk sac are attached. It's involvement with embryo and its function can just be seen by gently removing the entire contents of an egg into a Petridish and remaining the intact structure. This membrane and its contents serve to protect the embryo against the physical damage and also function as an area of exchange. As the embryo enlarge, the membrane stretches to accommodate the increase in size and serve less and less in the role of buffer against physical motion. By the time the embryo has hatched, the membrane is thinly stretched and barely visible as its surrounds to fully developed form.

Selecting Eggs for Virus Propagation

1. Determination of Viability of egg- The viability of embryo and the progress of embryo development is determined by candling. The egg at interval during incubation candling consist of giving the egg against the constructed light source preferably in dark room so that the shadow of embryo and associated structure, specially blood vessels are visible for routine purpose, it is necessary to candle the egg only on the day of use to establish that the embryo has reached the normal size and is alive. Generally the healthy embryo shows the characteristics movement & will impart an orange yellow colour to its egg because of blood circulating in vessel. In embryo which is dead or dies will have low, no; or sluggish movement and will be easily detached because of the diminish of vessel or their complete absence. If the embryo has grown large enough nearly to fill the egg lack of motion may be only due to death: An egg obtaining a small embryo (dead) will usually have a cleared yellow colour. Any colouration tending to green or black is an indication of extreme contamination and such egg should be carefully removed and placed in a discard container. In addition the content may have consistency of water rather than the viscous character of an healthy egg. Candling also enables in selecting point of entry through the shell. The point should not be situated directly over the large blood vessels adhering to the underlying shell membrane. As any puncture in them during inoculation may lead to haemorrhage and death of embryo. The point of inoculation and air space should be marked at the time of egg candling.
2. Sterilization of egg - Egg shell is sterilized with the swab tightly squeezed in tincture of iodine, taking care that not too much of the solution soak into the shell. Alternatively 70% ethyl alcohol may be used .
3. Age of embryonating egg and suitability to various inoculation route - The age of embryo best suited to propagation of virus and route of inoculation as worked out should be used. Little success follow it attempts are made substitute the route of inoculation.
4. The age of embryo and route of inoculation commonly employed for propagation is shown in table.

Table Route of inoculation in embryonated eggs

Route of inoculation	Age of embryo	Volume of inoculum	Viruses for which used
Chorio allantoic route (CAM)	10-12	0.1	Fowl pox, pigeon pox, vaccinia, herpes simplex, herpes zoster, infectious laryngotracheitis, pseudorabies
Allantoic cavity	9-12	0.1	Ranikhet disease virus, infectious bronchitis, influenza virus , mumps, eastern, western, Venezuelan equine encephalitis virus, para influenza.
Amniotic cavity	7-15	0.1	Influenza virus, mumps virus
Yolk sac	5-8	0.1	Blue tongue virus, mumps virus
Intravenous	10-15	0.01	Blue tongue virus
Intracerebral	8-14	0.01	Herpes simplex, rabies

Piercing the shell

The size of opening necessary for inoculation varies considerably depending on the route employed and for this purpose, the dental drill is suitable. With this type of device, simple holes may be cut with an ordinary drill attachment, while whole segment may be cut from shell with a rotating carborandum disc. The segment are then removed gently piercing of with a sterile scalpel whatever the size of opening; the actual drilling process should cut through the shell only leaving the underline shell membrane intact; the latter must never be pierced by drill.

Techniques of embryo inoculation

The methods of inoculation are as follows:

1. Allantoic sac inoculation
2. Amniotic sac inoculation

3. Yolk sac inoculation
4. Chorioallantoic membrane (CAM) inoculation
5. Intraembryonic
6. Intracerebral
7. Intravenous

The first four methods are in common use will be described briefly. The other three methods require considerable experience and skill to perform and are limited to special work.

A) Allantoic sac inoculation

Materials - Embryonated 9-10 days incubated eggs, inoculum or virus suspension, tuberculin syringe with 27 gauge ¾ to 1 inch needle, rubber cork with a pin, egg candler, rubber bulb, tincture iodine, molten wax, etc.

Procedure

1. Candle the egg and mark the boundary of air sec with pencil.
2. Select an area of the chorioallantoic membrane free of large blood vessels about 3 mm below the base of the air sac.
3. In this area make a pencil mark at the point for inoculation and other mark on air sac.
4. Apply tincture of iodine at the sites selected for making holes.
5. Rubber cork with a pin dipped in tincture iodine is used for making holes on the air sac as well as on other selected site.
6. Using a 1 ml tuberculin syringe fitted with a needle through a hole in the side of egg to a depth of about 1/4 inch and deposits the inoculum.
7. Withdraw the needle and inoculate the next egg or keep the syringe in sterile tube from where it was removed.

For use of 0.1 ml or more of inoculum the hole over the air sac is a necessary air vent to accommodate the inoculum within the egg and to prevent the inoculum from escaping through the hole on the side of the egg.

1. Seal the holes in the eggs with molten wax.

Amniotic sac inoculation Procedure

1. Candle 12-13 days old egg and make a pencil mark on the shell below the base of the air sac to locate the embryo.
2. Draw a circle parallel to and above 5 mm, above the base of air sac.
3. Using a small corborundum disc cut through the shell at the circle but do not pierce the shell membrane.
4. Apply tincture iodine to the groove cut by the disc and allow to dry.
5. Using forceps, remove the cap of shell over the air sac to expose the shell membrane.
6. Apply a few drops of sterile saline solution to the shell membrane over the embryo to make the membrane transparent. To cover more than about % of the shell membrane will interfere with the respiration and may result in the death of the embryo.
7. Using a 1 ml tuberculin syringe fitted with a 27 gauge, 1 inch needle, insert the needle into the amniotic cavity and inject the inoculum.
8. Close the opening in the shell over the air sac by sealing a disc of sterile heavy paper to the shell with molten wax.

C. Yolk sac inoculation Procedure

1. Candle 5-7 days old egg and mark the position of embryo and yolk sac.
2. Apply tincture iodine and disinfect the site of inoculation.
3. Drill a small hole through the shell at the upper extremity of the shell over the air sac.
4. Use a 20-22 gauge 1% inch needle and insert it perpendicular through the hole to the depth of at least 1 inch and deposit the inoculum.
5. Seal the hole in the egg with molten wax.

D) Chorioallantoic membrane (CAM) inoculation

Procedure

1. Candle 10-12 days old egg and make a pencil mark on the shell below the base of the air sac. Then, select a site on the side of embryo about 3 mm above & parallel to the base of the air sac for making the hole without puncturing the CAM.
2. Mark the second site for making hole over the air sac. Apply tincture iodine on both the sites.
3. Make the hole on both the sites taking care not to puncture the CAM with the help of rubber cork containing small pin.
4. For producing an artificial air sac over the CAM, air is sucked with the help of rubber bulb from the hole in air sac. Thus, air will pass through the opening made over embryo side permitting the chorioallantoic membrane to drop from the shell membrane at this point. The embryo membranes and fluid will fill normal air sac, thus creating an artificial air sac on the side of egg.
5. Using a 1 ml tuberculin syringe with a 27 gauge, Y_2 inch needle, insert the needle through the shell membrane over the artificial air sac and deposit the inoculum on the CAM.
6. Seal the holes with molten wax.

Post inoculation procedure - Sealing

The egg is sealed immediately after inoculation to prevent desiccation and maintain sterility. Simple drill holes are readily sealed with a piece of adhesive tape which is water proof and needs no sterilization before use. Large "windows" in the shell are best sealed with paraffin wax and a glass coverslip. A shoulder of wax is first built up round the neck, which is then covered with paraffin wax and a glass coverslip; a shoulder of wax is first built up round the hole which is then covered with a warm, sterile cover subsequent cooling of the glass serves to seal the hole.

Incubation Temperature - The optimum temperature for the development of the embryo (38-39°C) is too high for proper replication of most viruses and incubation temperature is accordingly reduced during the post incubation period to about 37°C, the exact temperature depending upon the virus being studied. The lower temperature has no significant effect upon the embryo during the few days. It is usually under observation.

Humidity and air circulation

The same strict precautions concerning humidity of 65% during the pre-inoculation period also observed after the egg has been inoculated. Forced air circulation by fan should be available to insure balanced temperature distribution throughout incubation.

Position of egg

The position of the egg after inoculation depends upon the location in the shell of the largest aperture. The later must remain uppermost, so that there is the least risk of the egg content being lost. Thus, after inoculation by the amniotic route the egg is incubated in a horizontal position. Contrary to the pre-inoculation procedure; the egg must not be turned at any time after inoculation.

Examination schedule

Inoculated egg should be candled with same frequency until determination made concerning length of time necessary to observe the length of the inoculation. Examine eggs after 18-20 hours but never late then 24 hours. The examination is to find which are dead or dying from trauma of inoculation. Some eggs may die within the time period due to virus inoculation. The death of embryo within 24 hours are un-specific, so eggs should be discarded.

Total duration of candling period can be determined by:

1. Nature of virus
2. Response pattern of embryo
3. Tissues/cell harvested

For example, yolk is to be harvested the embryo should be removed before 12th day of incubation. The surviving embryo should still be examined for death or gross pathology. Changes initially candling for examination for eggs can be continued until hatching time but practically 15th day of inoculation until can be seen. Because of the increased size of embryo and hence, opacity.

❑❑❑

Experiment **4**

Preparation of Media and Reagents for Cell Culture

The cell cultures became commonly used after the introduction of antibiotics and fungistatic substances, the use of laminar flow cabinets is also very helpful in preventing the contamination of culture as well as the leakage of virus. However, the aseptic precautions are still essential. The finger contamination is possible and this necessitates careful handling of cell culture material. There are antibiotic resistant mycoplasmas, which pose problem. The cultured cells are used for virus isolation, virus titration, vaccine production and biochemical studies. Since 1949 when Enders, Weller and Robbins reported that poliovirus could be grown in non-neural cells with the production of cytopathic changes, large number of unknown viruses were isolated in cell cultures. The advantages of cell culture over chicken embryos or experimental animals are:

1. Cell cultures can be produced in large quantities and stored at -70°C.
2. Cell cultures give a clear cytopathic effect.
3. Cell cultures can be grown in chemically defined medium, which is free from antibodies or other infections.
4. Cell cultures can be radiolabelled to study the details of virus multiplication.

Preparation of solutions

Phosphate buffered saline (PBS)

Solution A

Sodium chloride	8.0 gm
Potassium chloride	0.2 gm

Disodium phosphate	1.15 gm
Monopotassium phosphate	0.2 gm
Glass distilled water	800 ml

Solution - B

Calcium chloride	0.1 gm
Glass distilled water	100 ml

Solution C

Magnesium chloride 6 H_20	0.1 gm
Glass distilled water	100 ml

Mix solutions A, B and C together and sterilize in autoclave

2. Hanks balanced salt solution (HBSS)

Sodium chloride	8.0
Potassium chloride	0.4
Calcium chloride	0.14
Magnesium sulphate	$7H_20$ 0.1
Magnesium chloride	$6H_20$ 0.1
Disodium phosphate	$2H_20$ 0.06
Monopotassium phosphate	0.06
Dextrose	1.0
Phenol red	0.02
Sodium bicarbonate	0.35
Triple glass distilled water	1000 ml

Added in the form of 0.4 per cent solution

To be added before use on form of 1.4 per cent solution.

For 1000 ml of Hanks BSS, 5 ml phenol red solution (0.4%) and 25 ml of sodium bicarbonate solution (1.4%) is required. Therefore, dissolve the ingredients in a total volume of 970 ml distilled water.

For preparing this, take 500 ml distilled water in a flask and put the ingredients after weighing them in the order mentioned. Dissolve completely each of them before putting the next ingredient. After dissolving all the ingredients, bring the volume to 970 ml by adding 410 ml distilled water, then add 5 ml phenol red solution. Now the total volumes becomes 975 ml, this may now be distributed in 97.5 ml aliquots and sterilized. At the time of use, appropriate amount of sodium bicarbonate solution is added (2.5 ml of sodium bicarbonate solution to 97.5 ml of HBSS). Antibiotics are added at the time of use.

Hanks balanced salt solution without phenol red

This solution is the same as the previous one except that phenol red is omitted. It is required when medium is prepared for agar over day technique for viruses. This facilitates the staining of the over day with neutral red or any such dye.

Calcium and magnesium free hanks solution

The ingredients are the same as listed for hanks solutions except that contains calcium and magnesium ions. This solution is used for preparing the trypsin solution in order to enhance cell dissociation during the trypsinization process.

Calcium and magnesium free saline

Glucose	1.0
Sodium chloride	8.0
Potassium chloride triple glass	0.4
Distilled water	1000 ml

Dissolve the ingredients in the order mentioned. This solution is required for preparing trypsin solution where calcium and magnesium ions are required.

Trypsin (0.25%)

One gram trypsin (TC;Difco 1.250) is dissolved is 400 ml of calcium and magnesium free solution and is stirred on magnetic stirrer either at 4°C for overnight or at room temperature for 30 minutes. After this the solution is Seitz filtered and kept at 20°C in aliquots.

Phenol Red (0.4 or 1%)

One gram or 0.4 gram phenol red is taken in a pestle and mortar and triturated with small amount of N/5 NaOH solution till it completely dissolves after which the volume is made to 100 ml with triple glass distilled water. It is filtered through what man No. 42 filter paper and sterilized at 15 lbs pressure for 15 minutes.

Calf Serum

Blood from heating cow calf is collected and kept in the refrigerator at 4°C. Over night the lot is formed and serum is separated which is then collected, then it is kept at room temperature (25°C) for about 1 to 2 hours after which the serum is collected. Now it is centrifuged at 3000 rpm for 30 minutes to remove the red blood cells, if facilities are available, the centrifugation should be carried out in the refrigerated centrifuge to maintain the good quality of the serum and prevent haemolysis of erythrocytes. The serum is then inactivated at 56°C for 30 minutes seitx filtered and stored at 20°C in aliquots after testing for its sterility.

Horse serum

Methods of collection and preparation of the serum are the same as described for the calf serum. In many cell cultures horse serum is used, when it is suspected that the caly serum might contain some antibodies against the virus, which is being cultivated.

Preparation of Media Growth Medium

The commonly used growth medium for primary cell cultures, such as bovine kidney, lamb kidney, etc. is lactalbumin hydrolysate yeast extract (LAH-YE) growth medium. It consists of the following:

Lactalbumin hydrolysate (Difco TC)	0.5 gm
Yeast extract (Difco Bacto)	0.1 gm
Hanks balanced salt solution	80 or 90 ml

The solution is sterilized by seitz filterization or autoclaving at 10 lbs for 10 minutes. Then, the following ingredients are added:

Calf serum	10 or 20 ml
Penicillin	100 unit per ml

Streptomycin	100 ugm per ml
Mycostatin	25 unit per ml
Sodium bicarbonate solution (1.4%)	2.5 ml

The total volume of the medium should come to 100 ml, therefore, the serum and antibiotics are added to make the volume upto 100 ml.

The final pH of the growth medium should be 7.4. For kidney cell culture, serum is used at the rate of 20 per cent while embryo fibroblast and testis culture 10 per cent is used. For cell lines, 20 per cent serum should be used. The pH of the medium should be checked with the help of pH indicator paper (BDH). If the pH is less, add few drops of sterilized sodium bicarbonate solution. If pH is more, then bring it down by adding few drops of dilute hydrochloric acid.

Maintenance Medium

The constituents are the same as listed for the growth medium except that serum is either omitted for added is 2.5 per cent concentration. In case of foot and mouth disease virus work, no serum is added.

Siman Virus (S.V) Antiserum

SV5 and SV40 viruses are common contaminants of Rhesus monkey tissue even though the tissue is obtained from apparently healthy animals. When cell culture from monkey is prepared, SV5 and SV40 antisera should be incorporated in the cell culture medium to supress them.

Synthetic Media

Primary cell culture can grow in a good growth medium containing lactalbumin hydrolysate, yeast extract and calf serum or any other suitable serum in balanced salt solution. However, diploid cell strains and permanent cell lines require more nutritional ingredients e.g. several vitamins and aminoacids and thus, media incorporating these ingredients are required. Such media which contain all the nutritional requirement in the form of synthetic ingredients are called as synthetic media. These media are prepared from ingredients whose chemical purity is well known. The commonly used media are listed below:

- Medium 199
- Eagle's minimum essential medium.
- Eagle's basal medium
- RPMI -1640
- Ham's F-12
- BHK 21, Medium

These media are now commercially available in the country in powder form. They are dissolved in triple glass distilled water and NaHCCb, antibiotics, and serum are added and sterilized by seitz filtration.

The addition of serum (10-20) is done as per the requirement of the cell line, some cell line, such as BhK2, require 1-glutamine and this amino acid is added additionally while preparing the medium. Similarly, tryptose phosphate broth may be added for better growth and maintenance of the cell line, some of the cell lines require foetal calf serum.

HEPES Buffered media

If HEPES (N-2 hydrony ethyl piperazine - N-ethane sulphonic acid) buffered medium is to be sued where CO2 incubators are not available, then HEPES should be used in 20-25 mm concentration along with 10 mm $NaHC0_3$, when earls base is used. The composition of a representative HEPES buffered growth medium for a BHK21 cell is as follows:

Trypton phosphate broth	2000 mg
L-glutamine	300 mg
HEPES	4760 mg
$NaHC0_3$	850 mg
BHK21, medium (powder) with earls base	1000 ml
Distilled water	1000ml
Calf serum	100ml

In the maintenance medium the serum may be reduced to 2-5% or avoided altogether, when working with apthovirus.

Preparation of Cell Culture

There are three types of cell culture as defined below:

- Primary cells
- Primary cells populations are cells obtained from intact animal tissues and grown on glass or plastic surface for the first time.

Diploid cell strains

Diploid cell strains are primary cell populations that have been subcultivated several time which retain the normal chromosomes constitution of the tissue of origin, and are capable of a finite number of subcultivation.

Heteropioid cell lines

Heteroploid call cell lines are cell populations that can be sub-cultivated indefinitely, which reveal abnormal chromosomes number or morphology, and posses abnormal chromosome number or morphology, and possess other properties that distinguish them from normal cells.

Primary Cell Cultures

Tissue obtained from neonatal or young animals can be used to obtain large quantities of cells. Although these cells do not have long life *in vitro*, they are highly suitable for virus isolation since the various types of cell present in the primary culture ensure a wide spectrum of sensitivity to viruses while the established cell lines may have a narrow spectrum of viruses to which they are susceptible since embryonic or young tissue cells are capable of undergoing more multiplication cycle *in vitro* as compared with cells from adult animals, the age of the animal should be as low as possible. The requirement and susceptibility to viruses for primary cell culture is shown in table.

Table Primary cell cultures, their media requirement and sensitivity to viruses

Primary human Embryonic kidney	Eagle's MEM with 10% bovine serum	Epith	Polio, rhinovirus, measles, mumps, entero virus, herpes
Primary rabbit kidney	Eagle's MEM with 10% bovine serum	Epith,	Wide variety of viruses rubella, herpes B, required for testing of all human vaccines produced in primary monkey kidney culture.
Primary bovine kidney	Eagle's MEM with 10% bovine serum	Epith, fib,	Bovine viruses such as FMD, P13, IBR, bovine virus diarrhoea.
Primary rat embryo	Eagle's MEM with 10% bovine serum	Epith, fib.	Viruses affecting rodents
Primary monkey kidney	Eagle's MEM with 10% bovine serum	Epith, fib.	Several human viruses, adenoviruses
Primary Hamster embryo	Eagle's MEM with 10% bovine serum	Epith, fib.	Adnovirus 12, herpes simplex, influenza A, reovirus
Primary chick embryo	Eagle's MEM with 10% bovine serum	Epith, fib.	Influenza, vaccinia, measles, NDV, poultry viruses
Primary lamb kidney	Eagle's MEM with 10% bovine serum	Epith	Sheeppox goatpox lumpy skin disease
Primary bovine thyroid	Eagle's MEM with 10% bovine serum	Epith	FMD
Primary bovine tasty	Eagle's MEM with 10% bovine serum	Epith	Viruses affecting bovines

Primary mouse embryo	Eagle's MEM with 10% bovine serum or medium 199	Epith, fib.	Viruses affecting mice
Primary chick kidney	Eagle's MEM with 10% bovine serum	Epith, fib.	Viruses affecting chicken

Epith = Epithelial, Fib = Fibroblastic

❏❏❏

Experiment 5

Subculture and Maintenance of Continuous Cell Lines

When the cell culture monolayer grown in bottles are subcultured into other bottles, they are called secondary cultures. Usually secondary cultures are better, when the cytopathic effect (CPE) and the inclusion bodies are to be observed by staining since the cells are spread up better as compared with the primary culture. In addition several tissues, such as bovine kidney, lamb kidney, monkey kidney, embryonic kidney, etc. are not easily available, it is advantageous to subculture, the primary culture to prepare secondary cultures so that additional bottles or tubes and cell suspension for microplates are available and more study can be done with the limited cells available.

1. Select a bottle having a complete monolayer and decant the medium.
2. Wash the monolayer with CMF - BSS Thrice.
3. Add 2 ml trypsin (0.25%) and spread on the monolayer surface by gentle rotation.
4. Decant the trypsin leaving about 0.5 ml in the bottle.
5. Incubate the bottle at 37°C for 1-5 min. Watch in between for the effect of trypsin on the monolayer. As the cells would become round due to the action of trypsin, adjust the time of incubation accordingly.
6. Decant the excess trypsin.
7. Add 10 ml growth medium and detach the cells by uniform pipetting examine the bottle under microscope for complete detachment of the cells.
8. Add sufficient volume of the growth medium so as to prepare three bottles. If desired, count the cells and make dilutions accordingly. Similarly, if desired, centrifuge the cells and again

resuspend so as to completely remove the traces of trypsin, the serum in the growth medium inactivate the trypsin and poses no problem.

9. Incubate at 37°C and observe for cell multiplication and monolayer formation.

Table. Established cell lines, their media requirement and virus sensitivity

Species	*Cell line*	*Derivation*	*Growth medium*	*Split ratio*	*Morphology*	*Viral susceptibility*
Cattle	MDBK	Bovine kidney	MEM, 10% fetal bovine serum (FBS), 2 mm glutamine	1:10	Fib.	BVD, IBR, VSV
	IMR-31	Buffalo lung	McCoy's 5A, 20% FBS, 2 mm glutamine	1:2	Fib.	HSV, vaccinia pseudorabies BVD, PI 3, IBR, bovine enterovirus, VSV
Hamster	BHK21/ Cl13	Polled kidneys from 1 day old syrian hamster	Eagle's MEM glasgow modified, 10% FBS, 2 mm glutamine, 10% tryptose phosphate broth	1:30	Fib.	FMDV, rabies, pseudorables, Adenovirus, VSV, reovirus, polyoma
Human	Hela	Cervical carcinoma	MEM, 10% FBS, 2Mm glutamine	1:40 Epith	Poliovirus, Adenovirus	
	HEp2	Carcinoma of larynx	Eagle's basal medium 15% FBS 2 mm glutamine	1:20	Epith.	Poliovirus, Adenovirus, VSV

	KB	Oral epidermoid carcinoma	MEM, 5% FBS, 2mM glutamine	1:20	Epith	Poliovirus, Adenovirus
	Flow-2002	Human embryonic lung	Eagle's basal medium 10% FBS, 2 mm glutamine, 1% non-essential	1:2	Fib.	Poliovirus, HSV, RS, sendai, Rhinovirus
Monkey	BSC-1	African green monkey kidney	MEM, 10% FBS, 2 mm glutamine	1:2	Epith.	Polio, VSV, SV40
	Vero	African green monkey kidney	Medium 199, 5% FBS, 2mM glutamine	1:15	Fib.	Semliki forest virus, tacaribe, herpes simplex
Mouse	Clone M3	Melanoma cloudman S91	Ham's F10, 2.5% FBS, 15% horse serum,3 mm glutamine	1:2	Epith.	HSV, vaccinia, VSV, pseudorabies
	NCTC clone L929	C3H/An mouse areolar and adipose tissue	Ham/s F10 2.5% FBS, 15% horse serum, 2mM glutamine	1:4	Neuroblast	HSV, VSV, vaccinia
	3T3	Swiss mouse embryos	Eagle's medium, dulbecco's	1:20	Fib.	Polyoma, HSV, vaccinia
	3T3	Swiss mouse embryos	Eagle's medium, dulbecco's	1:50	Fib.	HSV, VSV, pseudorabies

Cell Lines

The greatest advantage in using a cell line is that it gives an unlimited amount of cells by continues passages. The cell lines always grow uniformly and can be grown on glass or plastic surfaces as monolayer as well as in suspension. The subculturing of cell lines is done in the similar way as described for secondary cultures. The established cell lines, their media requirement and virus sensitivity are given in table.

Micro Cultures In this system, cells are grown in microtiter plates, which can be used for various purpose in virology, immunology, and serology. Its application has increased manifold and now it has become a routine procedure.

Micro Carrier Culture

Micro carrier culture is a culture system in which the tissue cells are grown as monolayers on the surface of small solid particles and kept suspended in the culture medium by constant stirring. In this way the characteristics of both suspension culture and monolayer culture are brought together while retaining all the advantages of both culture systems the micro carrier culture method provides an enormous growth surface area to volume ratio and by using micro carriers in simple suspension culture yields of several million cells per milliliter can be obtained. In this culture as in suspension culture, measurement and control of the environmental conditions, such as temperature, pH, O_2 and CO_2 tension are facilitated. In addition, replacement of the medium and washing of the cells are facilitated.

Suspension Culture

When a large yield of cells is required, the suspension culture is the best method. The cells are growth in suspension without allowing them to attach on the surface of the vessel and this is achieved by constant stirring of the vessel contents, the O_2, CO_2, pH and other environment conditions are provided to suit the requirement of the cells.

For cultivating cells on a moderate scale, a suitable vessel with a plastic enclosed magnet is available, and after adding the cell suspension the vessel is placed on a magnetic stirrer so that the cells are maintained continuously in suspension.

For suspension culture on a large scale, larger size fermenter vessels of several hundred litre capacity are employed with electronic controls for maintaining all the required optimum conditions. Suspension culture are mainly employed for the manufacture of vaccine.

❑❑❑

Experiment **6**

Quantitation of Cells by Viable Cell Counts in a Haemocytometer

Cells are suspended in PBS containing trypan blue and then examined to determine the percentage of cells that have clear cytoplasm (viable cells) versus cells that have blue cytoplasm (nonviable cells).The cells can be counted under light microscope using haemocytometer.

Clean haemocytometer and coverslip, wipe with alcohol before use. Moisten the coverslip with water and affix to the haemocytometer. The presence of Newton's refraction rings under the coverslip indicates proper adhesion.

Preparing cell suspension

1. Gently swirl the flask to ensure the cells are evenly distributed.
2. Before the cells have a chance to settle, take out 0.5 mL of cell suspension using a 5 mL sterile pipette and place in an Eppendorf tube.
3. Take 100 µL of cells into a new Eppendorf tube and add 400 µL 0.4% Trypan Blue (final concentration 0.32%). Mix gently.

Counting

1. Using a pipette, take 100 µL of Trypan Blue-treated cell suspension and apply to the haemocytometer. If using a glass haemocytometer, very gently fill both chambers underneath the coverslip, allowing the cell suspension to be drawn out by capillary action. If using a disposable haemocytometer, pipette the cell suspension into the well of the counting chamber, allowing capillary action to draw it inside.
2. Using a microscope, focus on the grid lines of the haemocytometer with a 10X objective.

3. Using a hand tally counter, count the live, unstained cells (live cells do not take up Trypan Blue) in one set of 16 squares (Figure 1). When counting, employ a system whereby cells are only counted when they are set within a square or on the right-hand or bottom boundary line. Following the same guidelines, dead cells stained with Trypan Blue can also be counted for a viability estimate, if required.
4. Move the haemocytometer to the next set of 16 corner squares and carry on counting until all 4 sets of 16 corners are counted.

Viability

To calculate the number of viable cells/ml

1. Take the average cell count from each of the sets of 16 corner squares.
2. Multiply by 10,000 (10^4).
3. Multiply by 5 to correct for the 1:5 dilution from the Trypan Blue addition.

The final value is the number of viable cells/mL in the original cell suspension.

Example : If the cell counts for each of the 16 squares were 50, 40, 45, 52, the average cell count would be:

(50 + 40 + 45 +52) ÷ 4 = 46.75

46.75 x 10,000 (10^4) = 467,500

467,500 x 5 = 2,337,500 live cells/mL in original cell suspension

To calculate viability - If both live and dead cell counts have been recorded for each set of 16 corner squares, an estimate viability can be calculated.

1. Add together the live and dead cell count to obtain a total cell count.
2. Divide the live cell count by the total cell count to calculate the percentage viability.

Example : Live cell count: 2,337,500 cells/mL

Dead cell count: 50,000 cells/mL

2,337,500 + 50,000 = 2,387,500 cells

2,337,500 ÷2,387,500 = 97.9% viability

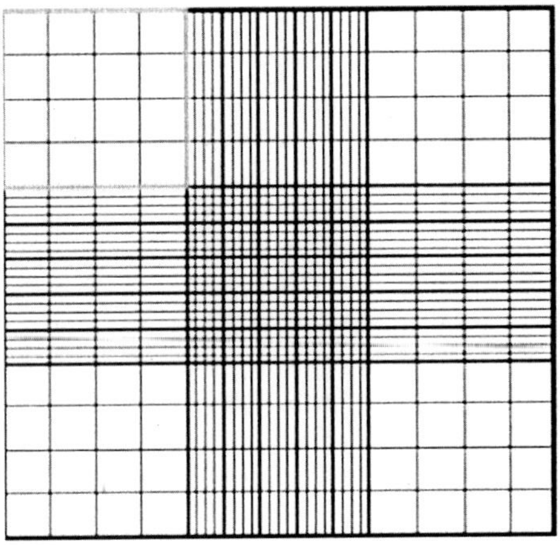

Figure: Haemocytometergridlines

Experiment 7

Cryopreservation and Recovery of Cell Cultures

Cells can be stored for an indefinite period in a frozen state under liquid nitrogen. To optimize freeze viability, use actively growing cells whenever possible; they are your insurance against accidental loss.

Composition

Cryoprotective solution; by volume:

Fetal bovine serum (FBS), 50%

Dimethyl sulphoxide (DMSO), 20%

Tissue culture medium, 30%

Method

1. Harvest the cells by centrifugation (150 *g* for 10 min at 4°C), count and adjust to 1×10^7/ml.
2. Add cell suspension dropwise to an equal volume of cryoprotective solution.
3. Dispense convenient volumes into ampoules suitable for storage in liquid nitrogen.
4. Freeze slowly (at about 10/min) down to at least –50°C and then immerse in liquid nitrogen.

Note:

i) DMSO (or alternatively, glycerol) allows water to go from a liquid to a solid state without the formation of ice crystals.

ii) Always use a fresh bottle of DMSO every 2–3 months to avoid the accumulation of toxic peroxides.

iii) DMSO must be handled with care: it can penetrate the skin and carry with it any harmful substance in regular use; for example, carcinogens.

Recovery of Cells

Cells may be recovered from liquid nitrogen storage by thawing rapidly to 37°C (in a water bath) and washing three times in tissue culture medium by centrifugation (150 *g* for 10 min at room temperature).

❑❑❑

Experiment 8

Preparation of Primary Cell Culture

(Chicken Embryo Fibroblast or Lamb Kidney Cell Culture)

Select a 10 days old fertile egg received from a disease free flock and incubated properly. Select only well-developed, active embryos with good blood supply, then candle the eggs and select a proper one.

1. Apply tincture iodine on the entire surface of the egg and keep the egg's air seal end uppermost.
2. With the help of sterile forceps, break the egg shell at the air sac, flame the forceps in between.
3. Remove the shell, the shell membrane and the chorioallantoic membrane.
4. Using the curved forceps take out the the embryo by catching it by the peak and place it in a petridish containing B.S.S. likewise remove several embryos using different sets of instruments.
5. Wash the embryo several times with BSS so that it becomes clean.
6. Using a pair of scissors and a forceps remove the head and limbs. Then, remove the internal organ by tearing the abdominal wall with the scissors.
7. Transfer the embryo to a beaker containing BSS and wash it several times with BSS so that the blood and other debris are removed.
8. Mince the embryo with the help of a pair of curved scissors.
9. Wash the minced tissue with BSS several times by pouring fresh BSS, shaking the beaker well, allow the tissue fragments to settle and then discard the supernatant.
10. Give a final washing with trypsin solution warmed before at 37°C.

11. Transfer the tissue pieces to a trypsinizing flask containing a teflon coated magnetic bar and pour sufficient amount of trypsin.
12. Place the trypsinizing flask on a magnetic stirrer and run it at a moderate speed.
13. After 15 minutes of trypsinization shut off the stirrer, allow the tissue fragments to settle, and then discard the supernatant which process will remove the toxic factors released from the tissue fragments.
14. Pour fresh trypsin solution and continue trypsinization for 30 minutes after which shut off the stirrer allow the tissue suspension in a centrifuge tube with a funnel gauze.
15. Carry out such trypsinization 2-3 times depending upon the requirements of the cells or till almost all the tissue fragments are digested.
16. Centrifuge the cell suspension at 1000 rpm for 10 min and give two washing with BSS and finally with the growth medium.
17. Suspend the cells in 100 ml growth medium.
18. Count the cells and adjust the cell density at 10^5 cells/ml.
19. Distribute the cells in cell culture vessels.
20. Incubate at 37°C in the incubator monolayer forms in about 3-5 days. If required, change the medium on the third day.

Lamb Kidney Cell Culture

1. Select young healthy kidney from slaughter house and immediately keep in container containing BSS.
2. Wash the kidneys several times with BSS.
3. Cut the cortical portion into small fragments.
4. Wash several times with BSS and finally with trypsin solution.
5. Transfer the contents to a trypsinizing flask and pour fresh trypsin.
6. Trypsinize for 10 min and discard the supernatant.
7. Again pour fresh trypsin and trypsinize for 30 min, collect the dispersed cells in a centrifuge tube by passing the cells through a gaurge layer. Make two or three collections.

8. Centrifuge, preferably in a refrigerated centrifuge, the cell suspension collected above at 1000 to 15000 rpm for 10 min. Re-suspend the cell pellet in the growth medium without serum and again centrifuge. Thus, give two washings and finally re-suspend the cells in a measured volume of growth medium containing serum so as to give a final concentration of about 5 x 10^5 - 10^6 cells per ml, this may be achieved by counting the viable cells in a hemocytometer after trypan blue staining or approximately dilute the cell 1:250 to 1:300 (V/V/) by packed cell volume (PA/) of the cells.
9. Dispense the above cell suspension glass vessels of different size and volume depending upon the requirement of the culture. Use the type of vessel shown in table. Allow roughly 1:10 ratio of tissue cell suspension volume and the internal volume of the vessel to provide sufficient oxygen and ideal environment for the cells to grow.
10. Incubate the vessels at 37°C by keeping them flat (bottles, flasks) or in an inclined position (tubes in cell culture racks) or on a roller drum (bottles and tubes), run at a speed of 11-12 rpm observe the cultures after 24 hours under inverted microscope and daily thereafter for formulation of cell monolayer. Usually a confluent monolayer is formed in 4-6 days. Change the growth medium on the third or fourth day, if necessary.

Vessels used for cell culture

Vessels (glass or plastic)	**Volume of cell suspension to be dispensed**
15 x 125 mm culture tube	1 ml
petri dish (30 mm diameter)	2 ml
160 ml milk dilution bottle	10 ml
50 ml flask	5 ml
100 ml flask	10 ml
1 roux flask	100 ml
Microtiter plate	0.05 ml/well

□□□

Experiment 9

Demonstration of Cytopathic Effect by Viruses in Cell Culture

Cell culture fluid is assayed by this technique for presence of virus. Table shows the sensitivity of cell cultures for various viruses.

Table Cells culture suitable for isolation of viruses from clinical specimens

Aphthovirus (FMD Virus)	HEK, HeLa, Hep,2 BHK 21, PK 15, bovine thyroid, IB-RS2, bovine kidney
Bovine enterovirus	Calf kidney, monkey kidney, pig kidney, BHK 21
Vesicular exanthema	Embryonic tissue culture of pig, horse, dog, cat
EEE	CEF, lamb kidney, rhesus kidney, Vero, HeLa, Rabbit kidney, MEF, BHK21.PK15
WEE	Calf, lamb, rabbit, rhesus kidney cells, HeLa, MEF, BHK 21, PK 15, IBRS-2
VEE	Chick kidney, rhesus kidney, Vero, HeLa, hamster kidney, BHK 21
Japanese encephalitis	Vero, HeLa CEF, hamster kidney, BHK 21, pig kidney cell lines
Bovine virus diarrhoea	Bovine kidney, fetal skin, cat kidney, swine kidney
Swine fever (Hog cholera)	Swine kidney, swine testis, bone marrow, spleen, lymph-node, pig kidney
Equine herpes type 1	Primary rabbit kidney
Bluetongue	Bovine and bovine embryonic kidney and testis, chang liver, HeLa, BHK 21, L929
Vaccinia	RK 13, Vero CEF

❑❑❑

Experiment **10**

Demonstration of Titration of Virus by $TCID_{50}$ and Plaque Assay in Cell Cultures

It is often necessary to know the amount of infectious, i.e. viable, virus in solid tissues, in suspensions prepared from them, in blood or other body fluids, or in cell culture fluids. For example, in the usual form of neutralization test serum, or dilutions of serum, must be mixed with a fixed and known quantity of infectious virus. Again, in the preparation of vaccines, it is necessary to know the amount of attenuated virus present in each dose of a live modified vaccine; similarly virus for "killed" vaccines is usually titrated prior to inactivation so that the quantity of virus present is specified.

Two main techniques are available for titration, these being:

1. Quantitative

Estimation of the number of "lesion-forming" infectious units. These may be plaques forming units (PFUs) as assayed on cell cultures or pock forming units assayed on the chorio-allantoic membrane (CAM). This method gives the greatest accuracy but is often laborious and more difficult to perform than the quantal technique.

2. Quantal

Estimation of the theoretical quantity of a virus suspension, which would infect 50% of susceptible hosts of a given kind. This is a statistical abstraction comparable to an LD_{50} for a non-viable toxic agent. The unit is called a TCD_{50} or $TCID_{50}$ if estimated in cell cultures, and EID_{50} in eggs or an ID_{50} in animals. In this response the quantitative change e.g. death of animal, death of developing chick embryo, production of CPE in cell culture, is taken as the lessons or response of the virus inoculation.

Both techniques commonly require the preparation of a series of regular dilutions, e.g. 10-fold, 5-fold or 2-fold, of which known volumes are inoculated into susceptible host systems, e.g. 4 or more tube cultures or animals for estimation of an ID_{50}, 4 or more eggs for pocks on the CAM.

The differences are as follows:

- The "lesions-counting" methods involve an actual count of the number of virus-specific foci present on the CAM or a monolayer inoculated with one suitable dilution of virus. These foci must not be too numerous or too small to count accurately and they must not merge with one another - this would introduce subjective errors. Their number should be great enough to limit sampling errors.
- In the 50% endpoint method, a record is made of the number of infected and non-infected hosts in each group inoculated with a number of dilutions which span the range 100% infected to nil infected.

Calculations

Quantal assay

The quantal type of assay is the ratio of positive response to total number of possible responses. It is employed into 50% end point method of titration and expressed as TCID (50% tissue culture infective dose), ID (50% infective dose), LD (50% lethal dose), as the case may be. For cell culture, it is numerically scored as shown below:

0 = No CPE

1 = 25% of the culture affected

2 = 50% of the cell culture affected

3 = 75% of the cell culture affected

4 = 75% to 100% of the cell culture affected

The results are expressed as a fraction in which the denominator represents the number of possible response and the numerator of observed responses. If 5 cell culture tubes are used per dilution, the maximum response would be 20, the sum of the positive scored for each of the five tubes per dilution is 12, the result for the dilution would be recorded as 12/20.

The 50% endpoint by the Reed and Muench (1938) method is determined as explained in table.

Table: Reed and Muench procedure for interpretation of 50% end points

		Dilution of virus			
		10^{-6}	10^{-7}	10^{-8}	10^{-9}
	Positive rates	20/20	10/20	3/20	0/20
Accumulation Totals	Positive response	20	10	3	0
	Negative response	0	10	17	20
	Positive	33	13	3	0
	Negative	0	10	27	47
	Positive rates	33/33	13/23	3/30	0/47
	% positive	100	56.5	10	0

In this example, the dilution which would be expected to be 50% positive response lies between 10^{-7} and 10^{-8} dilutions.

The proportionate distance between these two dilutions is inferred according to the following formulae :

$$\text{Proportionate} = \frac{\text{\% positive above 50\%} - 50}{\text{\% positive above 50\%} - \text{\% positive below 50\%}} \text{distance}$$

$$= \frac{56.5-50}{56.5-10} = 0.14$$

Log lower dilution (dilution in which positive next above 50%) = 7.0 Proportional distance (0.14) x log dilution (10) = -0.14

- Sum (50% endpoint) log $TCID_{50}$ = -7.14
- If 0.1 ml was used as inoculum, then $TCID_{50}$/ml = 10 x 10^{714} = 10^{814}
- With the karber (1931) method for 50% endpoint.
- Log $TCID_{50}$ = m-df[(s) - 0.5]

Where,

- M = log dilution containing highest concentration of virus Df = log of dilution factor
- S = sum of actual proportion of positive response to each inoculation,
- 0.5 = constant
- Using data in Table, the following is obtained :
- Log $TCID_{50}$ = -6 - (1.0) [0.15 + 0.5 + 1.0) - 0.5] = -7.15]

Virus titration in cell culture

1. Make 10-fold dilutions of the virus in tubes.
2. Take a pre sterilized 96-well flat bottom microtitre plate and add 50 µl of each dilution in two wells.
3. Add 50 µl of culture medium in each well keeping two wells as control in which no virus has been added.
4. Add 50 µl of cell suspension containing 10-cells/ml in each well.
5. Shake the plate and put the lid.
6. Incubate in CO_2 incubator with 5% CO_2 for appropriate time interval.
7. Remove the plate and dip formal crystal violet solution (0.1% crystal violet in 10% formalin saline). (While the infected and killed would have been lysed, the uninfected cells would take up the stain).
8. Examine the wells of each dilution. The highest dilution which shows 50% CPE is the dilution containing 1 TCID dose of virus. If this happens between two dilutions, determine the 50% end point using the Reed and Muench or the Karber method. Multiply by 20 to find out the TCID/ml in the original suspension.

Virus titration in developing chick embryo

There are several routes of inoculation of virus material in the developing chick embryo and the effect of virus on the embryo, e.g. death of the embryo, thickening of the CAM, etc., are recorded. The titer is expressed as LD (50% lethal dose) or ID (50% infective dose) and calculated by the Reed and Muench method as described above.

Virus titration in animals

Several viruses can be titrated in animals and the infectivity titer can be calculated. For example, aphthovirus can be titrated in suckling mice, guinea pigs, and cattle as described below:

Mouse assay

1. Prepare 10-fold virus dilutions in PBS.
2. Inject 0.05 ml of each dilution intraperitoneally into each of 6-8 suckling mice (5-7 days old).
3. Record mortality upto the sixth day after inoculation.
4. Express the virus titer as 50% mouse lethal dose (mouse LD).

Guinea pig assay

1. Prepare 10-fold virus dilutions in PBS.
2. Inject 0.2 ml of each dilution intradermopad (intraplantar route) into both hind footpads of each guinea - pig (0.1 ml per pad) using 5 guinea - pigs per dilution.
3. Record for production of primary lesions (on the inoculation site) and secondary lesions (for footpads, tongue) up to the fifth day after inoculation.
4. Express the virus titer as 50% guinea pig infective dose GP-ID).

Cattle assay

1. Prepare 10-fold virus dilutions in PBS.
2. Inject 0.1 ml of each dilution on 5 sites per dilution intradermo-lingually.

   Four dilutions may be inoculated in each tongue.

3. Record the lesion at 24 and 48 hr after inoculation.
4. Express the virus titer as intradermolingual 50% infective dose (IDL-ID50).

Enumerative (Quantitative) Assay

In this method, the number of pocks on CAM or plaques in cell culture in fluid medium or under agar overly are counted.

Pock assay

This can be used for all the viruses, which produce pocks on CAM of developing chick embryo.

1. Take 10-12 days old embryonated eggs.
2. Paint the entire surface of the eggs with 70% alcohol.
3. Candle the eggs and mark the well-developed CAM area devoid of blood vessel.
4. With the help of the electric drill remove a triangular portion of the shell from the marked area. Drill a hole on the air sac.
5. With the help of a rubber bulb suck the air from the air sac so that CAM is dropped from its shell membrane attachment at the triangular area.
6. Make serial 10-fold dilutions of the virus in PBS and inoculate 0.1 ml on the dropped CAM using 3-5 eggs per dilution.
7. Seal the opening with tape and incubate at 37°C in a humidified incubator for appropriate time depending upon the virus being assayed.
8. After incubation is done, remove the shell overlying the artificial air-space created.
9. Carefully remove the CAM and transfer to a petri dish containing 10% formal saline and count the pocks.
10. Determine the infectivity titer as described for plaques produced in cell culture and express as pock forming units per millilitre.

Plaque assay with agar overlay

The technique described is for kidney cell. With appropriate medium modifications, the same technique may be used for monolayers of almost any other type of cell.

1. Prepare confluent kidney monolayers in petri dishes or bottles.
2. Decant the growth medium completely.
3. Add 10 ml of Earle's saline lactalbumin hydrolysate standard pH, serum free maintenance medium to each monolayer, and incubate at 38°C for about 60 min. This is done to leach excess serum from the culture.
4. Aspirate the leaching fluid as completely as possible.
5. Prepare serial 10-fold dilutions of virus in Earle's saline - lactalbumin hydrolysate medium, and inoculate 0.1-ml volume of appropriate dilution directly on each monolayer. Inoculate two plates or bottles per dilution.
6. Incubate the infected monolayers at 37°C for 60 min to allow adsorption of virus to take place. Rock gently at 15-min intervals in order to distribute the inoculum evenly.
7. Set the plates or bottles on an accurately levelled surface.
8. Carefully add 10 ml of Earle's saline - calf serum nutrient agar, equilibrated at 45°C to each monolayer, and allow to set. (This procedure must be done in subdued light).
9. Monolayers in bottles: After closing, incubate in an inverted position in the dark at 37°C Monolayers in petri dishes: Incubate in an inverted position in the dark at 37°C in a humidified atmosphere at 5 per cent CO_2 in the air.
10. Count the plaques after 3-5 days incubation, when they appear more or less circular, pale areas on a pinkish background.

Staining and counting of plaques

Plaques are produced when the virus infects the cells and kills them. Thus, the monolayer may be stained in two ways: (i) Staining by a vital dye, e.g. neutral red which would stain the living cells leaving only the dead cells (plaques) unstained (ii) Staining by trypan blue which would stain only dead cells and thus, rendering the plaques clearly visible.

1. Staining of plaques with agar overlay intact.

One milliliter of 0.5% neutral red solution is put onto the agar overlay and incubated at 37°C for about 2 hrs after which the bottle or petri dish is inverted and further incubated for 4 hr. The bottle or petri dish is then transferred to the refrigerator (4°C) and kept overnight after which the plaques are counted. The bottle is placed on a carbon paper to provide a dark background and the counting is done is the oblique light.

2. Staining of plaques by removing the agar overlay

This method is good for petri dish cultures.

1. Take out the petri dish and put sufficient amount of absolute methanol to immerse the overlay.
2. Allow about 2 hrs and then decant the methanol and gently lift the agar overlay with the help of a forceps. Take out the whole overlay layer in this manner (Now the culture monolayer would be left over).
3. Give a final rinse with absolute methanol and decant it.
4. Put crystal violet or carbol fuchsin or trypan blue stain on the monolayer and let it remain for about 10 to 15 min.
5. Decant the stain and rinse with tap water to remove the extra stain.
6. Dry the petri dish and count the plaques. Preserve the petri dish for further demonstration.

Calculation of plaque forming units in virus suspension

The plaque forming units (PFU) per millilitre in a given virus suspension is calculated by the following formula:

N = VD

Where N = Titer as number of infectious units per milliliter

X = Average number of focal lesion

V = Volume of inoculum in millilitres

D = Dilution

In a series of dilutions differing by a constant factor, such as 2, the dilution will differ by a constant amount (log 1/2 = $10^{'03}$, log 1/4 = $10^{''04}$, log 1/8 = $10^{''0\ 9}$). If 0.5 ml of a 1/4 x 10~^{4} dilution of virus produced on the average 58.5 focal lesions, the inoculum volume being 0.5 ml (log $10^{'03}$), the titer N is:

N = 58.5 / (1/2 x 1/4x1 O$^{'4}$)

= 58.5 ($10^{'0\ 3}$x$10^{'\circ\ 6}$ x $10^{''0\ 4}$)

= 58.5/1 O$^{'49}$ = 5.7 x $10^{'6}$

Plaque assay with methylcellulose overlay

1. The procedure is the same as for agar overlay through the point of incubation after inoculation of the virus.
2. After the incubation the monolayer is washed 3 times with 10 ml warm PBS and covered with 10 ml of the medium containing 0.5 to 2.5% methyl cellulose. Double strength methylcellulose is prepared in distilled water, autoclaved, magnetically stirred in a 4°C refrigerator, and then added to an equal quantity of double strength medium.
3. The bottles are incubated for appropriate period at 37°C and then cooled to 4°C.
4. The methylcellulose is decanted, and the monolayer is washed 3 times with distilled water.
5. The bottles are fixed 2 hrs with 10% formalin, stained for 5 min with crystal violet 1:200 aqueous solution decanted, washed with tap water and air-dried before measuring and counting the plaques.

Plaque assay with fluid overlay

1. The procedure parallels the agar overlay to the point where the virus inoculation is done.
2. After this, the fluids are decanted and the cell sheets are washed twice with BSS.
3. Then, 10 ml of medium with antibiotics is added to each bottle. The bottles are stoppered, incubated at 37°C, and examined after appropriate interval for CPE and development of plaques.

4. The monolayers are fixed overnight by filling the bottles with 10% formalin, stained with crystal violet (1: 200 aqueous solution) for 5 min, decanted, washed with tap water, and photographed on a 35 mm film. The negatives are projected to obtain a 6.5 x enlargement. The plaques are traced on paper, counted, and measured.

Agar cell suspension plaque assay is an alternative assay specially suitable for those cells which do not form a compact monolayer and thus, when dealing with viruses which are to be grown in such cells, the agar cell suspension plaque assay is adopted. It has additional advantages that there is no need for preformed monolayers and freshly trypsinized cells may be used. Further, the virus and the cells do not come in contact with the glass and the toxic effects are eliminated.

Procedure

1. Take a 50-mm petri dish or flask or bottle.
2. Prepare the growth medium containing 1% agarose and keep at 48°C in a water bath to maintain it in molten state.
3. Pour 5 ml of the medium in each petri dish and allow it to solidify. (This well makes the basal agarose layer).
4. Make 10-fold serial dilutions of the virus being assayed.
5. Add 0.1 ml of each dilution of virus to 1 ml of freshly.
6. Trypsinized cells (2 x 10^7 viable cells/ ml) suspended in the growth medium and incubate at 37°C for 60-90 min for virus adosorption to cell.
7. Add 2 ml of the medium containing 1.5% agarose to the virus cell suspension. Shake the mixture gently to obtain even cell suspension.
8. Pour gently in an even layer over the already solidify basal layer and allow to solidify.
9. Incubate at 37°C for appropriate period depending upon the virus.
10. Stain with neutral red and count for plaques.
11. Calculate the virus titer as PFU/ml as described under plaque assay.

1. Microhemagglutination test Principle of the test

Many viruses possess the ability to adhere to the surface of red blood cells. This attachment is the result of the interaction between the virus particle and red blood cells. This property of the virus particle is utilized to qualify the virus concentration in a given virus suspension.

Collection of blood erythrocytes

1. Bleed the proper animal species with a syringe containing a small amount of Alsever's solution.
2. Remove the needle from the syringe and immediately place the blood in a bottle containing sufficient Alserver's solution so that a ratio of one volume of blood to four volumes of anticoagulant is used.

Preparation of erythrocytes

1. Rotate gently the bottle containing stock RBC and remove an aliquot in a graduated conical centrifuge tube. If debris is present in the blood, pass it through a layer of gauze or muslin cloth.
2. Wash the cells in PBS pH 7.2 three times at a speed of 900 g.
3. After the final wash, remove the supernatant. Then, remove the RBC with the help of 1 ml pipette and transfer the desired volume in PBS diluent. Fowl RBC is employed as 0.5% suspension and mammalian RBC as 0.4% suspension.

Phosphate-buffered saline, pH 7.2 (PBS)

Na_2HPO_4	1.096 ml/l
$NaH_2PO_4.H_2O$	315 ml/1
NaCI	500 ml/1
Distilled H_2O	1000 ml

This PBS should be used for washing RBC and for preparing and diluting all RBC suspensions, it is the diluent for the antigen in the HA test and for the antigen and serum dilutions in the HI test. It is also used in kaolin and RDE treatments of sera and should, in fact, be the only diluent employed anywhere in the standardized HA and HI procedure.

HI titre of serum is calculated for alpha procedure from the following formula:

$$\text{HI titer} = \frac{\text{Reciprocal virus end - point}}{\text{Reciprocal of serum end - point}} \text{x dilution of serum}$$

For example : From fig.

Reciprocal of virus endpoint = 512

Reciprocal of serum endpoint = 8

Serum dilution = 10

$$\text{HI titer} = \frac{512}{8} \text{x } 10 = 640$$

1. Take a microtiter U or V plate and dispense 25 μl of PBS into wells 2 to 12.
2. Dispense 50 μl of starting serum dilution (1/10) in well 1.
3. Prepare serial two-fold dilutions of the serum with 25 μl microdiluter.
4. Add 25 μl PBS to the control wells.
5. Dilute the pretitrated virus in PBS to contain 4 HA unit per 25μl
6. Dispense 25 μl virus suspension containing 4 HA unit per 25 μl to each well containing the serum.
7. Shake the plate manually or on microshaker, put the cover and allow it to stand at room temperature for 30 min.
8. Add 50 μl of the appropriate RBC suspension into all the wells.
9. Shake the plate manually or on microshaker and incubate at appropriate temperature.
10. Read for inhibition of the agglutination.

Result

❑❑❑

Experiment **11**

Demonstration of Neutralizing Antibodies by Serum Neutralization Test in Cell Culture

Equal amounts of virus and specific reference antiserum are allowed to react together and the reaction mixture is then inoculated into a susceptible test system (animal, chick embryo, or cell culture) which is observed for the sign of virus infection. The absence of any sign of infection indicates that virus infectivity has been neutralized, and serves to identify the virus agent. Alternatively, it helps in quantifying the amount of antibodies in a serum taking a known virus for the test.

Procedure

1. Constant virus varying serum method
2. Prepare 1/8 dilution of each serum and inactivate at 56°C for 30 min.
3. Prepare a two-fold dilution series of the above sera in a microplate using 50 µl microdiluters.
4. Add an equal volume (50 µl) of virus suspension containing 100 TCID 50 virus already titrated in microplates.
5. Incubate at 37°C for 60 min
6. Add 50 µl of appropriate cell suspension containing 1.5 x 10 cells per ml.
7. Seal the plates with adhesive tape and incubate at 37°C for appropriate time depending upon the virus.
8. Remove the plates and tip off the media into a bowl and dip the plates into the staining solution (0.1% crystal violet in 10% formal saline).

Result

The cytopathic effect would cause lysis of the infected cells and therefore, only the uninfected monolayer would fix and take up the stain. Virus neutralization is marked by the presence of residual areas of stained monolayers.

The highest dilution of serum showing more than 50% protection is taken as the endpoint titer. This may be calculated by the method of Reed and Muench (1938).

B. Constant serum varying virus method

1. Prepare 1/4 or 1/8 dilution of the serum.
2. Prepare a 10-fold dilution series of virus.
3. Add 50 μl of each dilution of virus to duplicate wells of the microtiter plate.
4. Add 50 μl of the diluted serum to each well.
5. Shake the mixture well and incubate it at 37°C for 60 min.
6. Add 50 μl of the appropriate cell suspension (susceptible to the virus) containing 1x10 cells/ml.
7. Seal the plate and incubate at 37°C for an appropriate time depending upon the virus.
8. Remove the plate, tip off the media, and dip it into the staining solution (0.1% crystal violet in 10% formal saline) for 30 min. Wash the plate with tap water and dry it.
9. Carry out simultaneous titration of the virus without serum.

Result

Find out the virus titer in control and the serum mixture tests using the Karber (1931) or the Reed and Muench (1938) method. For example:

Log virus titer in control test = 7.5 Log virus titer in serum test =4.5 Neutralization index (NI) =7.5-4.5 =3.0

Two Dimensional Microneutralization Test

1. Prepare a two-fold dilution of serum.
2. Prepare 0.5 log serum dilution of virus.
3. Dispense one serum dilution into one row, e.g. A to FI rows having 12 wells each. Thus, A row should be dispensed with say, 1/16 serum dilution, and B row with 1/32 serum dilution.
4. Dispense one virus dilution to two wells of each row. For example, well numbers 1 and 2 of each row (A to H) will receive one dilution of virus, and so on.
5. Keeps suitable control: serum control, virus control & healthy cell control.
6. Test each serum dilution by the above procedure against each virus dilution.
7. Take further steps as described in the procedure for the microneutralization test.
8. Take the observation and find out the 50% end point by the Reed and Muench or the Karber method for the antiserum titer, which is able to neutralize 10.25 and 10.1.5 TCID virus. Plot the observation on a graph paper and by interpolation find out the antiserum titer neutralizing the 10 TCID virus.

❑❑❑

Experiment **12**

Agar Gel Precipitation Test for Detection of Virus Infection

Agar gel immunodiffusion test (AGID)/Ouchterlony double immunodiffusion or passive double immunodiffusion. The immunodiffusion test is based on the ability of the antigen antibody complex to form a visible line of precipitate in an agar gel, when the antigen and the antibody meet after diffusion from separate points. The number of lines formed will depend upon the number of antigen antibody reactions taking place. It can be used to identify either antigen or antibody by using any one of the reagents, which is a known standard reference.AGID is the OIE referred test for diagnosis of Blue tongue disease.

Procedure

1. A molten 1% solution of agar in phosphate buffered saline is poured into a petri dish to give a layer of 2-3 mm thick, and allowed to set.
2. Circular wells of 2-4 mm diametre are cut into the agar so that each well is 5 mm away from its neighbour. In the simplest case, four wells are placed one each at the corners of a square.
3. The bottom of each well is sealed by adding, and rapidly removing, a small amount of molten agar.
4. Equal volumes of reference, unknown, and control reagents are then added to appropriate wells, and the petri dish is incubated in a humidified chamber at 37°C for a suitable period to allow diffusion and reaction to occur. The time required may be from a few hours to the whole night, depending upon the concentration of the reagents employed.

Results

A positive reaction between the antigen and the antibody is indicated by the appearance of fine lines of precipitate between the appropriate adjacent wells. The test may give three types of reactions: Reaction of identity, if two antigens are serological similar, precipitation line or bi-identical bands fuse completely. Reaction of non-identity, if two bands cross each other. Reaction of partial identity, if a spur is form with one of the arc.

❑❑❑

Experiment **13**

Titration of Newcastle Disease Virus by Haemagglutination Test

The heamagglutination test is used to quantify the amount of Newcastle disease virus present in a suspension.This is done by carrying out two-fold serial dilution of the viral suspension in a microtitre plate and then testing to determine an endpoint. This result can then be used to quantify the amount of heamagglutinin in the suspension and is expressed as a HA titre.

Materials required

- U/V bottom microtiter 96 well plate
- Single and multi-channel micropipettes =25 μl
- Chicken RBC =1 %
- Sample
- PBS/NS

Procedure

1. Dispence 25μl of PBS in each well of the microtitre plate.
2. Place 25μl of test sample in first well of first row. Sample are generally tested in duplicate or triplicate to minimise the error.
3. Use a multichannel pipette to carry out two-fold serial dilution across the plate until column 9.
4. Add 25 μl 1 per cent RBC to each well including column 10-12. the well in this column is control well that contain only PBS and RBC.
5. Mix properly by gently taping sides of the plate.
6. Allow the plate to stand for 45 minutes at room temp.

7. Read and record the results in each well. All the control well should be HA negative.

8. HA negative: means a sharp button of RBC at the bottom of the well.

9. HA positive: means a hazy films of RBC, no button of RBC at the bottom of the well.

10. Identify the end point. This will be the last well to show complete haemagglutination and contain one haemagglutinating unit. One HA unit in the haemagglutinin titration is the minimum amount of virus that will cause complete agglutination is the well that contain one HA unit.

Calculation of HA titre of the test sample

The HA titre is the reciprocal of the highest dilution that produce one HA unit.

If sample of NDV in 64 (1/64), dilution contains 1 HA unit.

The HA titre of the test sample will, therefore, be the reciprocal of $1/64 = 64 = 2^6$

So, the titre of the suspension of the ND virus can be expressed as 64 or 2^6 HA in 25 μl.

□□□

Experiment **14**

Haemagglutination Inhibition Test for Detection of Antibodies to Newcastle Disease Virus

Many viruses, such as myxovirus, togavirus, reovirus some enterovirus, adenovirus and pox-virus have the ability to agglutinate RBC of various species of animals, and this agglutination can be inhibited by immune serum specific for the infecting virus. This specific inhibition of haemagglutinating activity of virus by immune serum is known as haemagglutination-inhibition (HI). HI test are very specific and are of great importance in diagnosis of Newcastle disease virus. This is very simple, cheap, rapid and reliable. There are two procedures for performing HI test designated as alpha (constant-serum,diluted -virus) and beta procedure (constant-virus,diluted -serum) , the beta procedure is used most frequently in the laboratory.

Materials required

- U/V bottom microtiter 96 well plate
- Single and multi-channel micropipettes = 25 µl
- Chicken RBC = 1 %
- 2 or 4HA unit virus
- PBS/NS pH = 7.2

Method

1. Place 50µl of PBS in well 1-12 of first and second rows of the clean microtitre plate.
2. Add 50µl of normal serum to first well of first row. Mix serum and PBS of second well 5 times and transfer 50 µl to the third well . In this way make further serial 2-fold dilution of the serum till 12th well. Discard 50 µl of serum -PBS mix. from the 12th well.

3. Using separate tip prepare 2-fold dilution of anti-serum (heat inactivated) in wells of second row as prepared for normal serum above in (step 2).
4. Add 50 µl of virus antigen containing 4 HA unit (in 50 µl) to each well of first and second rows.
5. Add 50 µl of 1% RBC to all the wells.
6. Include serum control, RBC control and antigen control to establish specificity and sensitivity of the test.
7. Shake the plate backward and forward and from side to ensure an even suspension or RBC in the mix.
8. Incubate the test at room temp. and read after 20-30 minutes. Or until a clear pattern of haemagglutination has appeared in the controls.

Assesment

1. In serum containing HI antibody, there will be complete inhibition of agglutination of RBC. The HI titre is expressed as the reciprocal of the highest dilution inhibiting agglutination of the RBC.
2. The normal serum should not inhibit haemagglutination.
3. The HI titre of 2^5 or more is considered high tittered sera.
4. The serum control and RBC/PBS control should not agglutinate RBC, while virus control should agglutinate RBCs.
5. The end-point of the inhibitory activity of the serum is the highest dilution of the serum in which the agglutination is completely inhibited. The HI titer of the serum for the beta procedure is calculated from the following formula:

HI titer = Reciprocal of serum endpoint x number of HA units.

For example: If Reciprocal of serum endpoint = 80

Number of HA unit = 4, HI titer = 80 x 4 = 320

□□□

Experiment **15**

Elisa for Detection of Viral Antigen and Antibodies

Proteins and lipopolysaccharides can be passively adsorbed to the plastic has been exploited in the development of immunoassays (ELISA). Immunoassays involving the use of enzymes attached to one of the reagents utilized in the test can be termed as enzyme linked immunosorbent assay (ELISA). The resulting conjugate have both immunological and enzymatic activity. By having one of its components (Ag and Ab) labelled with an enzyme and bound to and immunosorbent support, the Ag-Ab complexes become immobilized. Subsequent addition of relevant substrate chromogen solution causes a colour change and such ELISA test can be read both visually and by spectrophotometer.

S.No.	Enzyme	Substrate
1.	Horseradish peroxidase (HRPO)	Ortho-phenylenediamine (OPD) and H_2O_2
2.	B-D galactosidase	O-nitrophenyl-D-galactoside(ONPG)
3.	Alkanine phophatase	P-nitophenyl phosphate

Types of Elisa

1. Direct ELISA
2. Indirect ELISA
3. Sandwich/trapping/capture ELISA
4. Competitive ELISA
5. Avidin-biotin ELISA
6. Liquid phase blocking ELISA

Direct ELISA using primary antibody protocol

Buffers and reagents

Bicarbonate/carbonate coating buffer (100 mM)

Antigen or antibody should be diluted in coating buffer to immobilize them to the wells:

3.03 g Na_2CO_3

6.0 g $NaHCO_3$

1000 ml distilled water

pH 9.6

PBS

1.16 g Na_2HPO_4

0.1 g KCl

0.1 g K_3PO_4

4.0 g NaCl (500 ml distilled water) pH 7.4.

Blocking solution

Commonly used blocking agents are 1% BSA, serum, non-fat dry milk, casein, gelatin in PBS.

Wash solution

Usually PBS or Tris-buffered saline (pH 7.4) with detergent, such as 0.05% (v/v) Tween 20 (TBST).

Antibody dilution buffer

Primary and secondary antibody should be diluted in 1x blocking solution to reduce non-specific binding.

General procedure

Coating antigen to microplate

1. Dilute the antigen to a final concentration of 20 μg/ml in PBS or other carbonate buffer. Coat the wells of a PVC microtiter plate with the antigen by pipetting 50 μl of the antigen dilution in the top wells of the plate. Dilute down the plate as required.

Test samples containing pure antigen are usually pipetted onto the plate at less than 2 μg/ml. Pure solutions are not essential, but as a guideline, over 3% of the protein in the test sample should be the target protein (antigen). Antigen protein concentration should not be over 20μg/ml as this will saturate most of the available sites on the microtiter plate.

Ensure the samples contain the antigen at a concentration that is within the detection range of the antibody.

1. Cover the plate with an adhesive plastic and incubate for 2 hrs at room temperature, or 4°C overnight. The coating incubation time may require some optimization.
2. Remove the coating solution and wash the plate three times by filling the wells with 200 μl PBS. The solutions or washes are removed by flicking the plate over a sink. The remaining drops are removed by patting the plate on a paper towel.

Blocking

1. Block the remaining protein-binding sites in the coated wells by adding 200 μl blocking buffer, 5% non-fat dry milk or 5% serum in PBS, per well. Alternative blocking reagents include blockACE or BSA.
2. Cover the plate with an adhesive plastic and incubate for at least 2 hrs at room temperature or, if more convenient, overnight at 4°C.
3. Wash the plate twice with PBS.

Incubation with primary and secondary antibody

1. Add 100 μl of diluted primary antibody to each well.
2. Cover the plate with an adhesive plastic and incubate for 2 hrs at room temperature.

This incubation time may require optimization. Although 2 hr is usually enough to obtain a strong signal, if a weak signal is obtained, stronger staining will often be observed, when incubated overnight at 4°C.

3. Wash the plate four times with PBS.
4. Add 100 μl of conjugated secondary antibody, diluted at the optimal concentration (according to the manufacturer) in blocking buffer immediately before use.

5. Cover the plate with an adhesive plastic and incubate for 1-2 hrs at room temperature.
6. Wash the plate four times with PBS.
7. Dispense 100 µl (or 50 µl) of the substrate solution per well with a multichannel pipette or a multipipette.
8. After sufficient colour development (if it is necessary) add 100 µl of stop solution to the wells.
9. Read the absorbance (optical density) of each well with a plate reader.

Sandwich ELISA

A sandwich ELISA measures antigen between two layers of antibodies (capture and detection antibody). The target antigen must contain at least two antigenic sites capable of binding to antibodies. Monoclonal or polyclonal antibodies can be used as the capture and detection antibodies in sandwich ELISA systems. Monoclonal antibodies recognize a single epitope that allows quantification of small differences in antigen. A polyclonal is often used as the capture antibody to pull down as much of the antigen as possible. Sandwich ELISAs remove the sample purification step before analysis and enhance sensitivity (2–5 times more sensitive than direct or indirect).

Coating with capture antibody

1. Coat the wells of a PVC microtiter plate with the capture antibody at 1–10 µg/mL concentration in carbonate/bicarbonate buffer (pH 9.6).

   Unpurified antibodies (e.g. ascites fluid or antiserum) may require increased concentration of the sample protein (try 10 µg/mL) to compensate for the lower concentration of specific antibody.

2. Cover the plate with adhesive plastic and incubate overnight at 4°C.
3. Remove the coating solution and wash the plate twice by filling the wells with 200 µL PBS. The solutions or washes are removed by flicking the plate over a sink. The remaining drops are removed by patting the plate on a paper towel.

Blocking and adding samples

1. Block the remaining protein-binding sites in the coated wells by adding 200 μL blocking buffer (5% non-fat dry milk/PBS) per well.
2. Cover the plate with adhesive plastic and incubate for at least 1–2 h at room temperature or overnight at 4°C.
3. Wash the plate twice with 200 μL PBS.
4. Add 100 μL of diluted samples to each well. Always compare signal of unknown samples against those of a standard curve. Run standards (duplicates or triplicates) and blank with each plate. Incubate for 90 min at 37°C.

Ensure concentration of standards spans the most dynamic detection range of antibody binding. You may need to optimize the concentration range to obtain a suitable standard curve. Always run samples and standards in duplicate or triplicate.

5. Remove samples and wash the plate twice with 200 μL PBS.

Incubation with detection and secondary antibody.

6. Add 100 μL of diluted detection antibody to each well.

Check that the detection antibody recognizes a different epitope on the target protein to the capture antibody. This prevents interference with antibody binding. Use a tested matched pair, whenever possible.

7. Cover the plate with adhesive plastic and incubate for 2 h at room temperature.
8. Wash the plate four times with PBS.
9. Add 100 μL of conjugated secondary antibody, diluted in blocking buffer immediately before use.
10. Cover the plate with adhesive plastic and incubate for 1–2 hrs at room temperature.
11. Wash the plate four times with PBS.

Detection

Horse radish peroxidase (HRP) and alkaline phosphatase (ALP) are the two most widely used enzymes for detection in ELISA assays.

Consider that some biological materials have high levels of endogenous enzyme activity (such as high ALP in alveolar cells, high peroxidase in red blood cells) that may result in non-specific signal. If necessary, perform an additional blocking treatment with levamisol (for ALP) or 0.3% H_2O_2 in methanol (for peroxidase).

ALP substrate

P-Nitrophenyl-phosphate (pNPP) is the most widely used substrate for most applications. Measure the yellow colour of nitrophenol at 405 nm after 15–30 min incubation at room temperature and stop the reaction by adding equal volume of 0.75 M NaOH.

HRP chromogenes

The substrate for HRP is hydrogen peroxide. Cleavage of hydrogen peroxide is coupled to oxidation of a hydrogen donor which changes color during reaction.

TMB (3,3',5,5'-tetramethylbenzidine)

Add TMB solution to each well, incubate for 15–30 min, add equal volume of stopping solution (2 M H_2SO_4) and read the optical density at 450 nm.

OPD (o-phenylenediamine dihydrochloride)

The end-product is measured at 492 nm. Keep and store the substrate it in the dark, as it is light sensitive.

ABTS (2,2'-azino-di-[3-ethyl-benzothiazoline-6 sulfonic acid] diammonium salt)

The end-product is green and the optical density can be measured at 416 nm. Always handle with care and wear gloves, as some enzyme substrates are considered hazardous (potential carcinogens).

□□□

Experiment **16**

Molecular Techniques for Viral Disease Diagnosis

Molecular biology techniques for the direct detection of viral genomes in the specimen will play an increasingly important role in the clinical virology laboratory in the 21st century. Molecular techniques can be divided into two categories: those that do not involve amplification i.e. hybridization with nucleic acid probes, and those that involve amplification e.g. PCR, LCR, NASBA, etc.

Nucleic Acid Probes

Nucleic acid probes are segments of DNA or RNA that have been labelled with enzymes, antigenic substrates, chemiluminescent moeities, or radioisotopes. They can bind with high specificity to complementary sequences of nucleic acid. Probes can be directed to either DNA or RNA targets and can be from 20 to thousands of bases long. The presence and the quantity of hybrids after hybridization is determined by the detection of the label. Probes are usually synthesized by one of the following three methods:

1. Oligonucleotide probes - these are usually less than 50 bases long and are synthesized chemically
2. PCR - will produce probes from 50 to several hundred bases long
3. Cloning - will produce probes several thousand bases long e.g. probe for complete HBV genome

Altering the stringency of the reaction will alter the sensitivity and specificity of the hybridization. Stringency relates to the number of mismatched base pairs that can be tolerated, when two nucleic acid molecules come together to form a double stranded molecule. Stringency is affected by several variables, including the temperature, salt concentration, and the pH of the hybridization reaction. High stringency is achieved by using buffers of low salt concentration or by conducting the hybridization reaction and stringency washes at higher temperatures. The higher the stringency of reaction, the less likely it is for mismatched base pairs to stay together.

The hybridization reaction may be carried out completely in solution phase, whereby both the target nucleic acid and the probe are free to interact in the reaction mixture. Solution hybridization has the advantages of being rapid to the carry and carry a higher sensitivity than solid phase hybridization. This is the approach taken by Abbott with their quantitative HVB-DNA assay. Nucleic acid bound to a solid surface are still available to participate in hybridization reactions. However, the sensitivity tends to be lower than that of liquid hybridization. However, this technique greatly facilitates the handling of multiple samples. The dot-blot and sandwich hybridization assays are commonly used in this respect. In situ hybridization assays, in which whole cells or tissue sections are put through the hybridization process has become an important research tool.

Despite having been around for many years, hybridization assays are still not in common use in the clinical virology laboratory. The main reason is that its sensitivity is not usually higher than far simpler conventional virological techniques, such as cell culture and viral antigen detection.

Polymerase Chain Reaction

PCR allows the in vitro amplification of specific target DNA sequences by a factor of 10^6 and is thus, an extremely sensitive technique. It is based on an enzymatic reaction involving the use of synthetic oligonucleotides flanking the target nucleic sequence of interest. These oligonucleotides act as primers for the thermostable Taq polymerase. Repeated cycles (usually 25 to 40) of denaturation of the template DNA (at 94°C), annealing of primers to their complementary sequences (50°C), and primer extension (70°C) result in the exponential production of the specific target fragment. Further sensitivity and specificity may be obtained by the nested PCR technique, whereby the DNA is amplified in two steps: In the first step, an initial pair of primers is used to generate a long sequence that contain the target DNA sequence. A small amount of this product is used in a second round of amplification, which employs primers to the final target DNA.

Detection of DNA sequence product of the PCR assay may be performed in several ways. The least sensitive and specific method is to size fractionate the reaction product on an agarose or acrylamide gel and stain the DNA with ethidium bromide. A more sensitive technique involves the attachment of DNA to a membrane through dot or slot-blot techniques followed by hybridization with a labelled homologous oligonucleotide probe. Alternatively, the PCR product may be probed directly by liquid oligomeric hybridization. However, these techniques provides no information on size of the amplified product and thus, could not exclude the possibility that the product originated from a region of the human genome which exhibits homology with the target CMV sequence. The most sensitive and specific detection methods result from combining the size information of gel electrophoresis with the improved sensitivity and specificity of hybridization techniques. This may be achieved by gel electrophoresis followed by Southern transfer and hybridization, or through liquid oligomeric hybridization followed by gel electrophoresis.

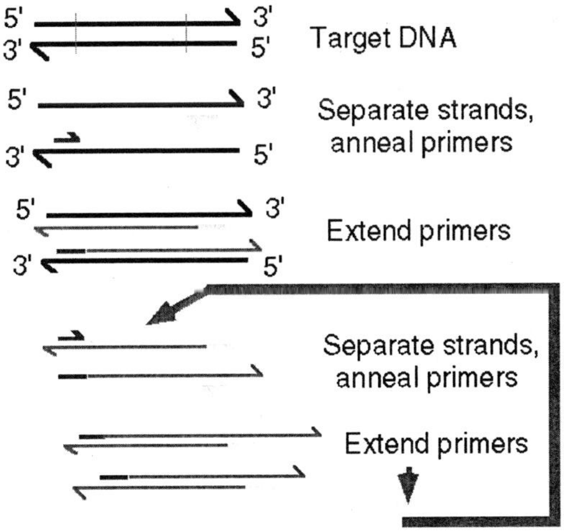

Schematic of Polymerase Chain Reaction

Advantages of PCR

1. Extremely high sensitivity, may detect down to one viral genome per sample volume
2. Easy to set up
3. Fast turnaround time

Disadvantages of PCR

1. Extremely liable to contamination
2. High degree of operator skill required
3. Not easy to quantitate results
4. A positive result may be difficult to interpret, especially with latent viruses, such as CMV, where any seropositive person will have virus present in their blood irrespective whether they have disease or not.

Real time quantitative PCR

In real-time PCR, the presence of the PCR product is monitored during the PCR process, not at its end. Real-time PCR can be used to quantify the PCR product. There are two common methods used in the detection of PCR product: non-specific fluorescent dyes and specific DNA probes. The fluorescent dye intercalate with any double-stranded DNA present. Whereas, the oligonucleotide DNA probes are labelled with a fluorescent reporter which permits detection only after hybridization of the probe with its target sequence e.g. the Taqman system. Real-time quantitative PCR is being increasingly used for viral diagnosis in routine laboratories.

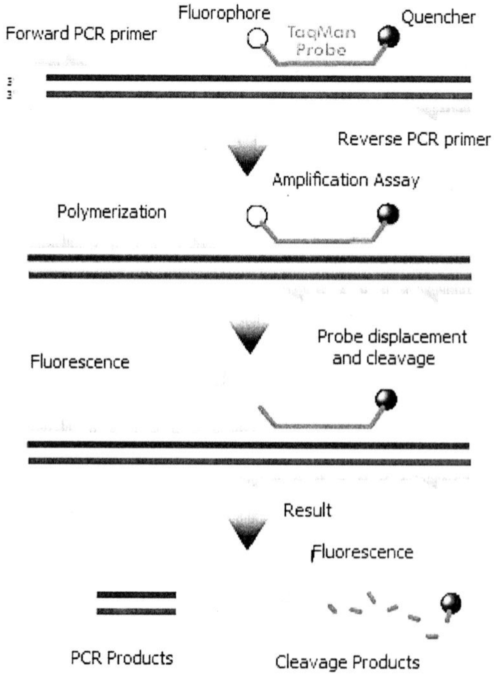

Other Amplification Techniques

Following the heels of PCR, a number of alternative in-vitro amplification techniques have been developed, of which some are now available commercially. Examples of these alternative techniques include ligase chain reaction (LCR), nucleic acid sequence based amplification/isothermal amplification (NASBA), strand displacement amplification, Q-Replicase method, and branched DNA probes. Of these techniques, LCR, NASBA and branched DNA are now available commercially in an automated or semi-automated format. A NASBA assay is available for the quantification of HIV-RNA (Organon), and an LCR assay is available for the detection of chlamydia (Abbott). Branched DNA assays are available for the detection of quantification of HIV-RNA, HBV-DNA, and HCV-RNA (Chiron).

With the exception of the branched DNA probe, all these techniques involve exponential amplification of either the target nuclei acid or the probe. Therefore, they are all as susceptible to contamination as PCR. The branched DNA system is really an intermediate between classical hybridization techniques and the newer in-vitro amplification techniques. It is not as sensitive as those techniques which involve exponential amplification but is considerably more sensitive than the classical hybridization techniques. Below is a brief summary of the features of the different amplification methods available.

Baltimore Classification of Viruses Based on Mode of Replication

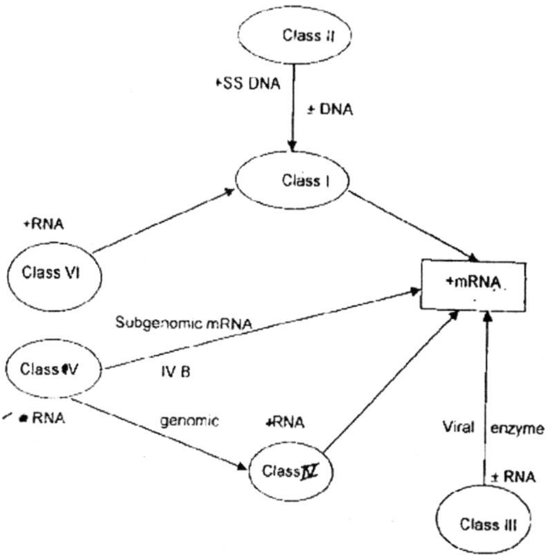

DNA viruses

dsDNA and enveloped

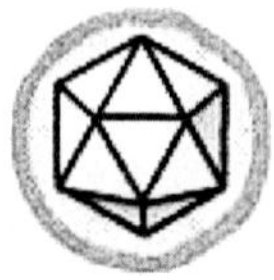

Herpesviridae

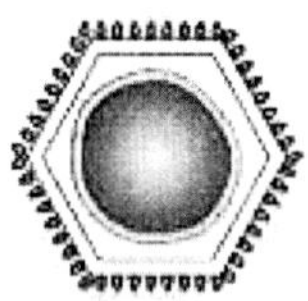

Asfarviridae

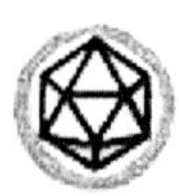

Hepadnaviridae

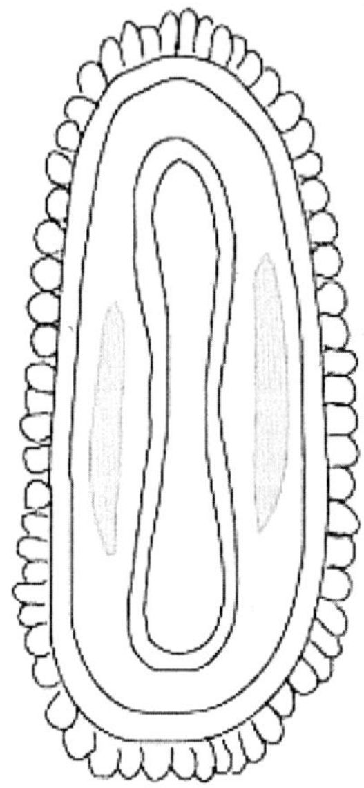

Poxviridae

dsDNA and non-enveloped

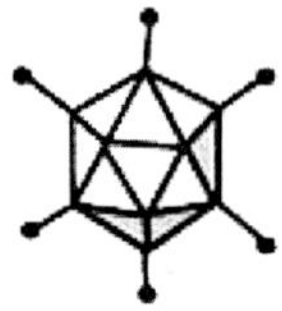

Adenoviridae

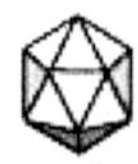

Papillomaviridae

ssDNA and non-enveloped

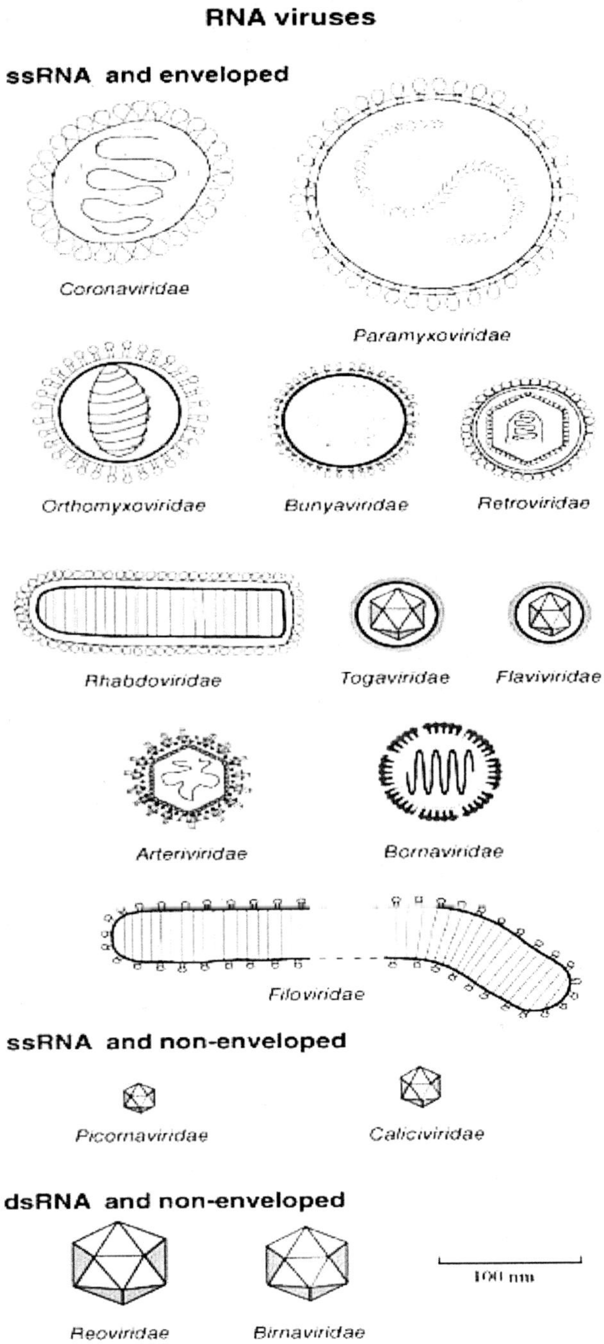
RNA viruses
ssRNA and enveloped
Coronaviridae
Paramyxoviridae
Orthomyxoviridae
Bunyaviridae
Retroviridae
Rhabdoviridae
Togaviridae
Flaviviridae
Arteriviridae
Bornaviridae
Filoviridae
ssRNA and non-enveloped
Picornaviridae
Caliciviridae
dsRNA and non-enveloped
Reoviridae
Birnaviridae
100 nm